Illustrative Atlas

Intralesional Bleomycin Injection (IBI) for

Hemangiomas and

Congenital Lymphatic Malformations

Mohamed A Baky FAHMY

Emeritus Professor of Pediatric Surgery

Al-Azhar University

For centuries, vascular birthmarks were referred to by vernacular names derived from traditional beliefs that a mother's emotions or patterns of ingestion could indelibly imprint her unborn fetus.

Hemangioma is the most common tumor in infancy, with a perinatal incidence of 1% to 2.6% with a rising incidence in the first year. They are speculated to affect 4% to 12% of white children. The exact pathogenesis is not well known.

Spontaneous epithelial breakdown, crusting, ulceration, and necrosis occur in 5% of cutaneous hemangiomas and are most common in mucosal hemangiomas of the lips or anogenital region.

The management of hemangiomas continues to be a subject of considerable controversy; surgery and different forms of laser should be kept for special cases, cortocosteroid injection could enhance involution of the hemangioma, and it was used long time ago, with a variable success. Recently the sclerotherapy with wide spectrum of medications was a treatment first option in such patients, it offering a viable alternative to surgery, especially in those affecting mainly the head and neck. Various agents, such as bleomycin, OK-432, alcoholic solution and doxycycline, and many other have been used for percutaneous sclerotherapy.

Lymphatic malformations (LMs)—traditionally known as lymphangiomas or cystic hygroma are benign vascular lesions caused by developmental disorders of the lymphatic system in the embryonic life. These lesions are most commonly found in the head and neck region (45–52% of all cases), which have significant propensity for appearing at birth and even prenatally. It is a consist of abnormally formed lymphatic channels and cystic spaces filled with eosinophilic and protein rich fluid. Based on the classification of the International Society of the Study of Vascular Anomalies, cystic LMs are divided into three categories: macrocystic, microcystic, and combined. LMs commonly appear as localized areas of cystic swelling which may be complicated by viral or bacterial infections, intralesional hemorrhage, inflammation, and/or trauma. Treatment options for LMs include resection, sclerotherapy, laser coagulation, and radiofrequency ablation, although some of these methods are often combined. Surgery is no longer a primary treatment option because it is difficult to perform complete excision without scarring, which is associated with recurrence or regrowth of the LMs.

The sclerosant agent damages the epithelial lining of cystic spaces, with a subsequent decrease in lymph fluid production and collapse of the cysts.

Bleomycin is well known as a cytotoxic antitumor antibiotic inducing DNA degradation, also it has a specific sclerosing effect on vascular endothelium, which was therapeutically used in the treatment of cystic hygroma and hemangioma with a significant response rate of 70% to 90%.

The authors presenting his own experience on management of 195 patients (105 hemangioma and 90 LMs) with different forms and different locations during the years from 1992 to 2024. Bleomycin was the first line of treatment for all cases.

Corticosteroids injection was tried for cases of hemangioma obstructing the respiratory tract or oral cavity to reduce the obstructive symptoms, but side effects are considerable.

Oral propranolol (Inderal) was tried only for superficial (Capillary hemangiomas) cases with a limited success, we reported some cases responding reversely with flourish and increase in size in response to oral inderal.

For hemangioma a 15 mg of bleomycin was diluted with 10 ml saline and administered by percutaneous injection according to age and size of the malformation by a hypodermic fine needle followed by local pressure. The patients received either a laryngeal mask or general anesthesia during the infiltration.

For large and deep lesions, the injection repeated ever 3 weeks. A total of 420 sessions were performed with an average total dose of 20 mg/m^2, in a single injection the dose calculated as 0.3–0.5 mg/kg, maximum single dose is 8 mg.

Local complications as infection and ulcerations were seldom seen, and no systemic toxic reaction was diagnosed.

Complete resolution was obtained in 75% of patients with much better results in cystic hygroma (80%) than in hemangioma (60%) or venous malformations (40%). Superficial capillary lesions are the least responders with 30% success. Usually, the large cavernous hemangioma and arteriovenous malformations are responding poorly to bleomycin injection, in such cases either a primary resection or resection after tissue expansion of the neighboring normal skin were indicated (10 and 9 cases respectively). Tissue expansion was used for 8 cases with a large and deep hemangioma of the abdominal wall.

Hemangioma and vascular malformations

1. Oral Inderal only effective in some cases of capillary hemangioma; face
    hemangioma before and six months after oral inderal.

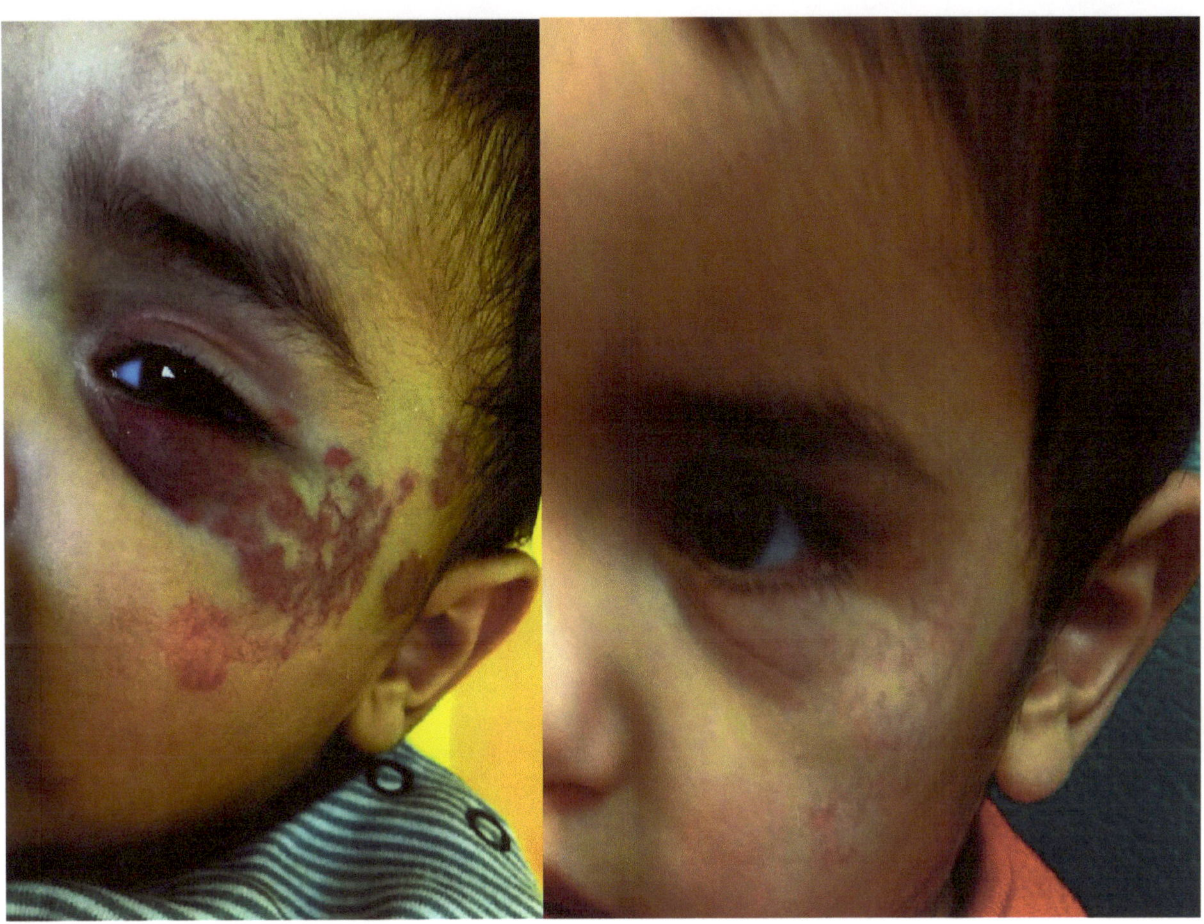

We have a limited experience with local injection of corticosteroids; and we used this modality mainly for infants with obstructive or compression manifestations to induce some relief of the swelling till the patient could be able to tolerate the bleomycin injection.

This one-year infant showed a limited response to local corticosteroid injection for an arm extensive hemangioma

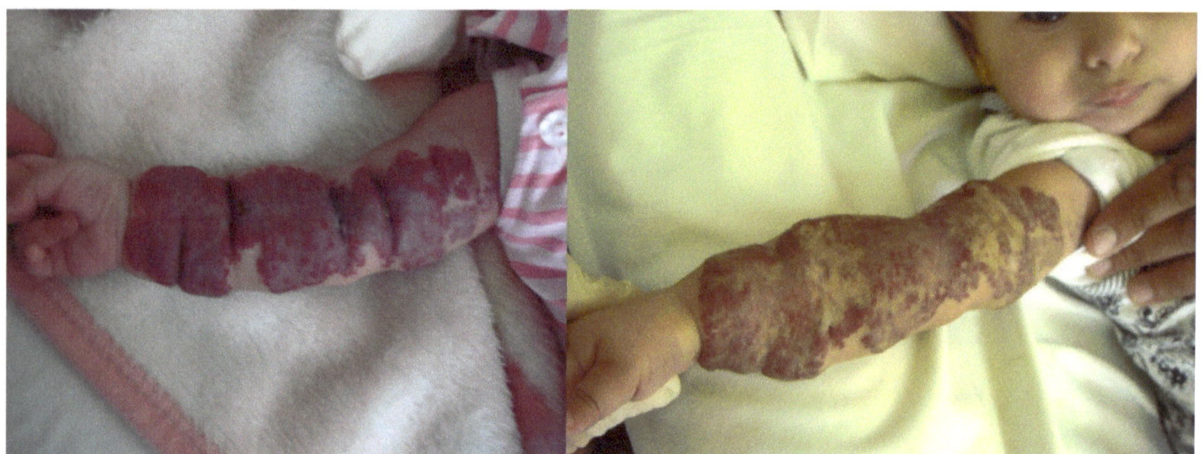

2. Inderal failure for leg combined hemangioma, in this cases even the oral Inderal induced flourish of the hemangioma, but there was an effective resolution after 6 sessions of bleomycin injection.

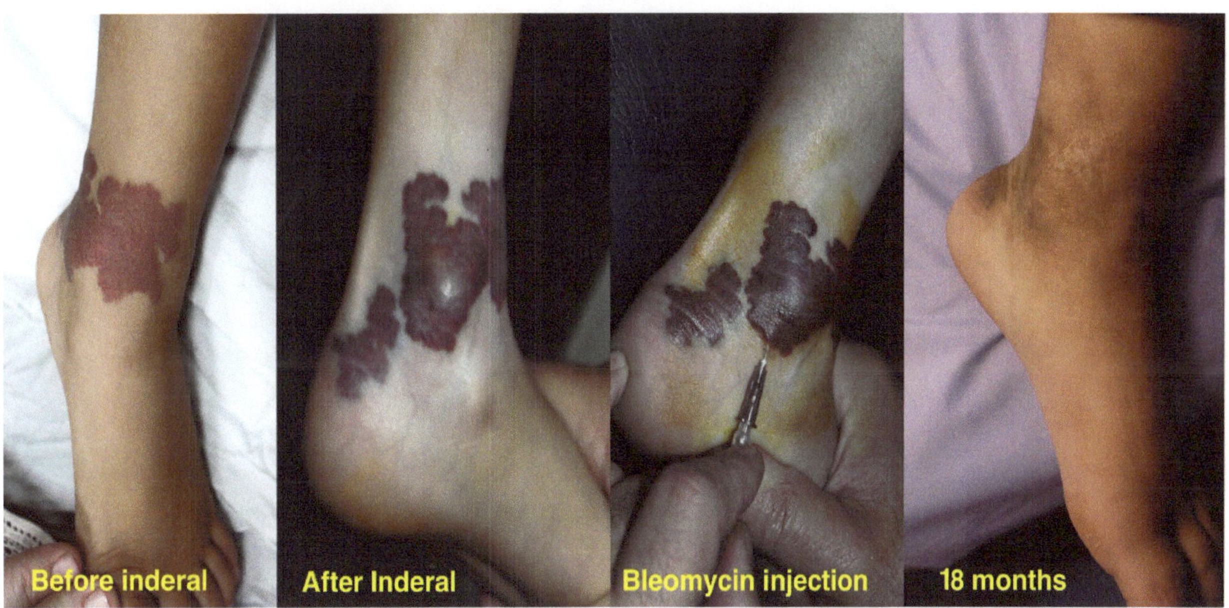

3. Cheek hemangioma with a partial response after 3 session of bleomycin injections

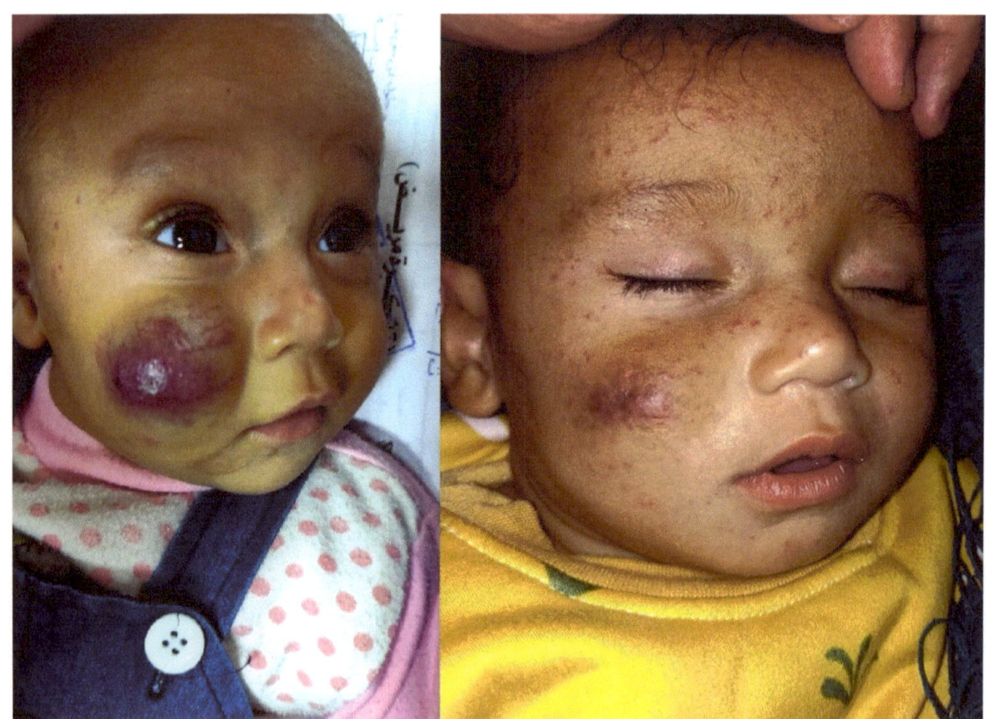

4. Cheek hemangioma with about 80% response after 3 sessions of bleomycin injections

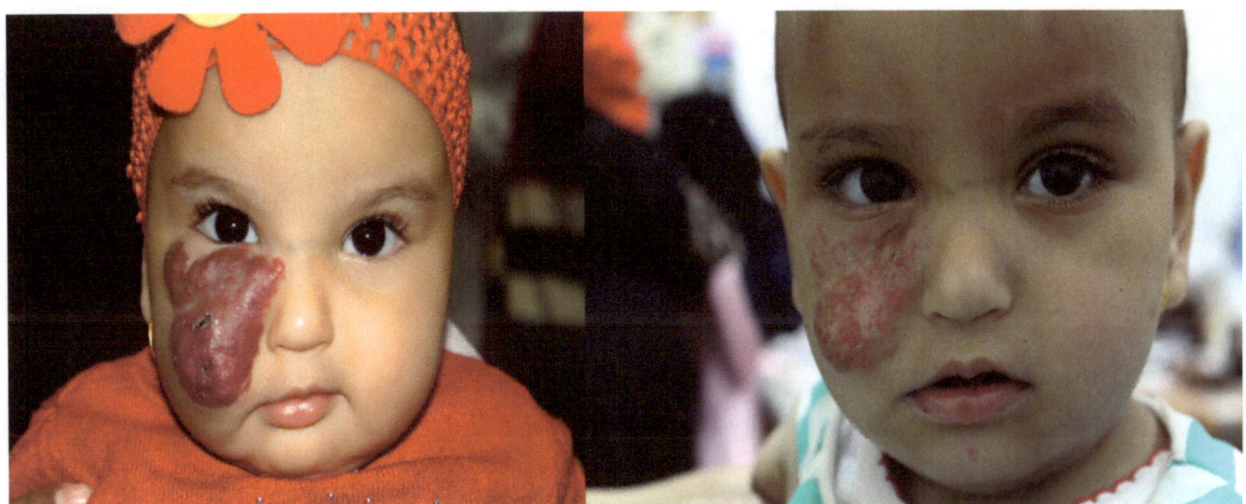

5. Upper lip hemangioma with a 100% resolution after 6 sessions of bleomycin injections

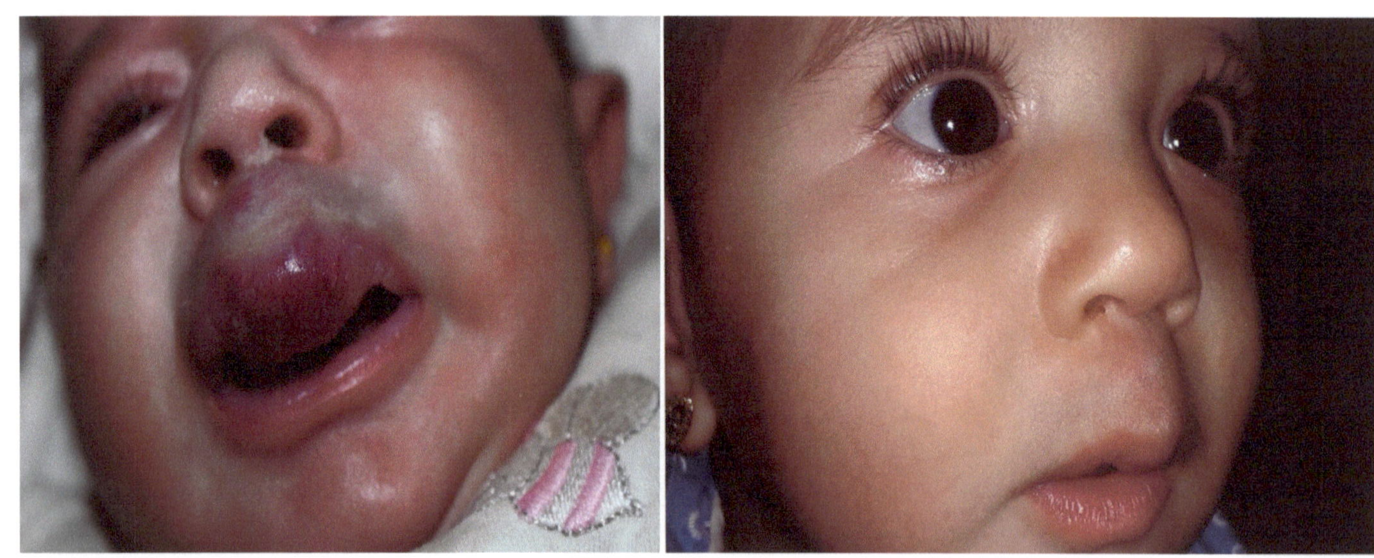

6. Huge upper lip cavernous hemangioma, complete resolved after 4 sessions of
    injections

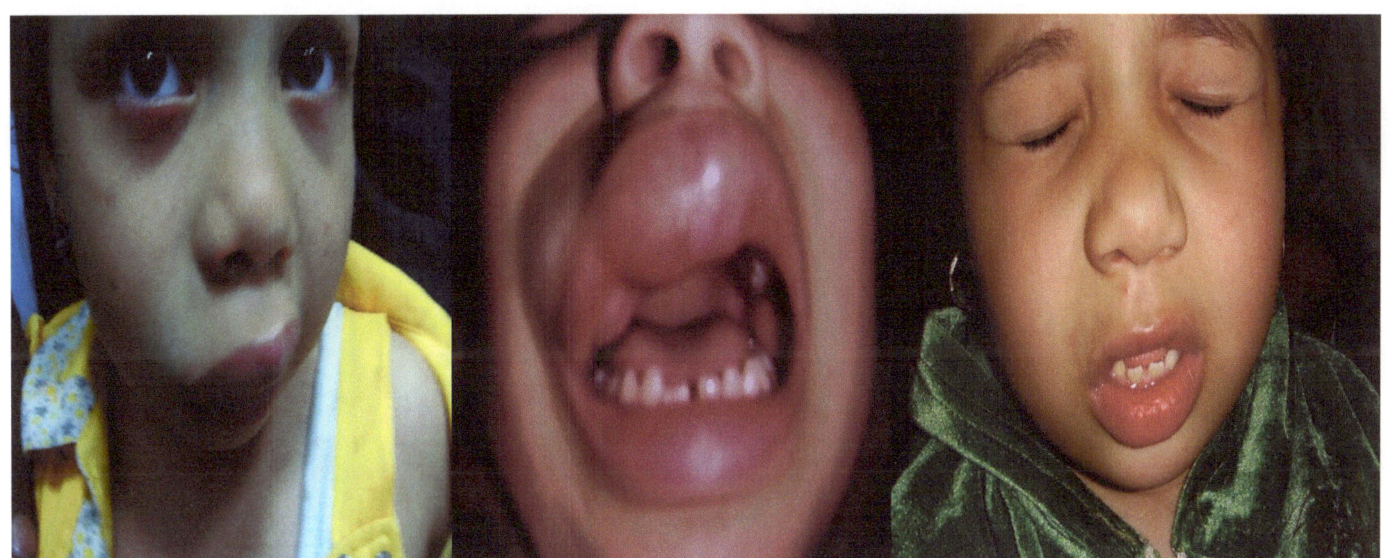

7. Upper lip combined superficial and cavernous hemangioma; residual
   cavernous component after 3 sessions, but the superficial component resolved
   completely.

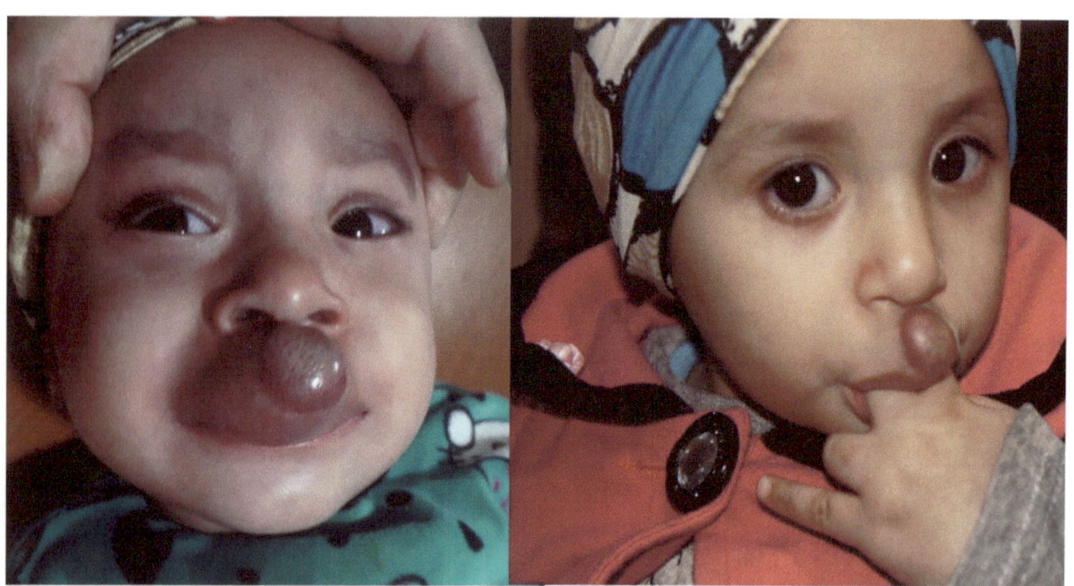

8. Extensive lower lip hemangioma resolved with some tissue loss after 6
    injections of bleomycin.

13

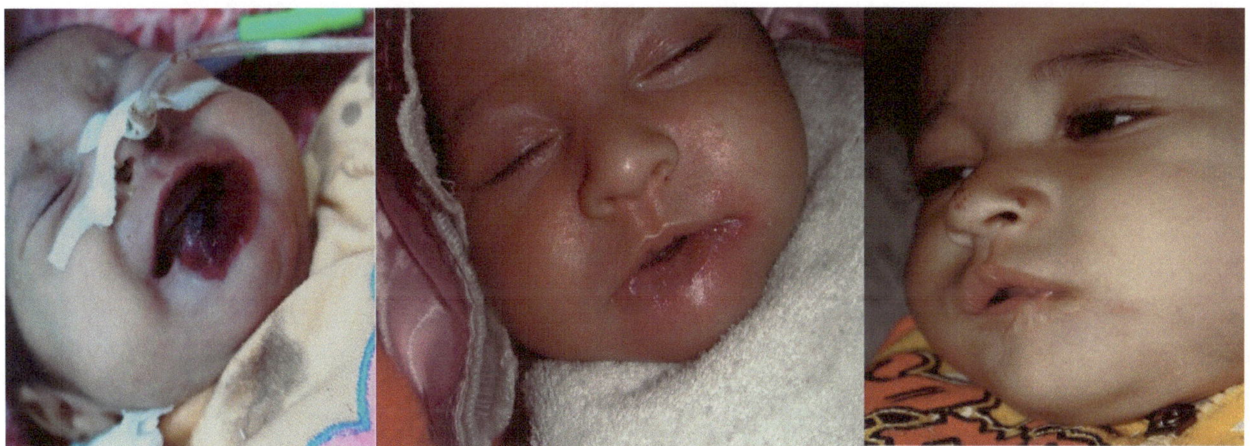

9. Lower lip skin loss after 5 sessions of bleomycin injection, but managed by
    bulking agent injection

14

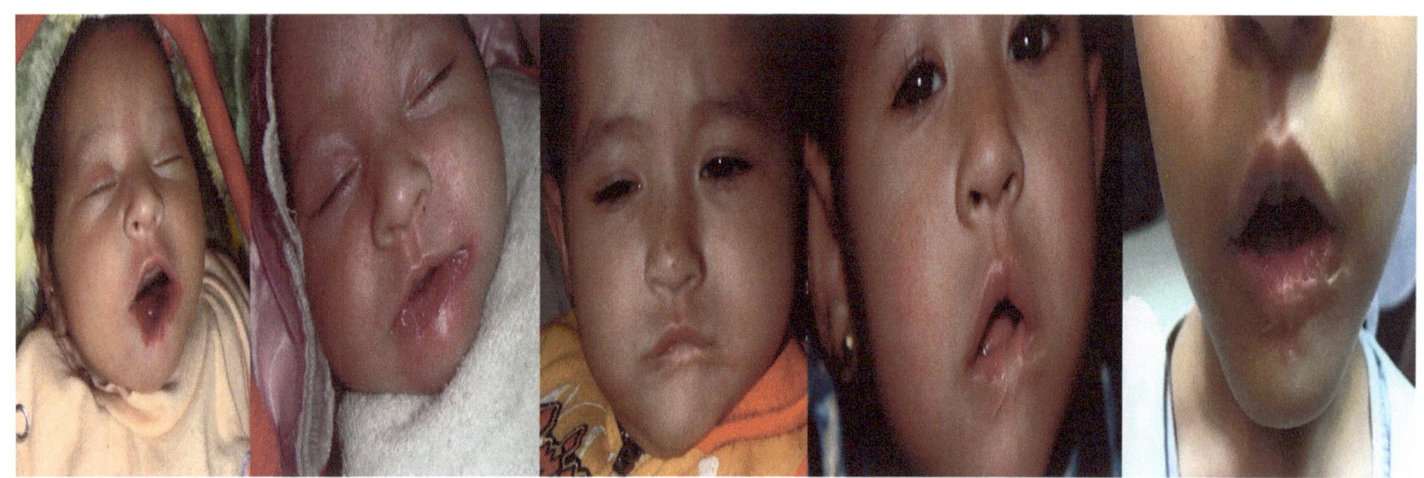

10.Inner lip hemangioma showed a complete resolution after 3 sessions of
   bleomycin injections

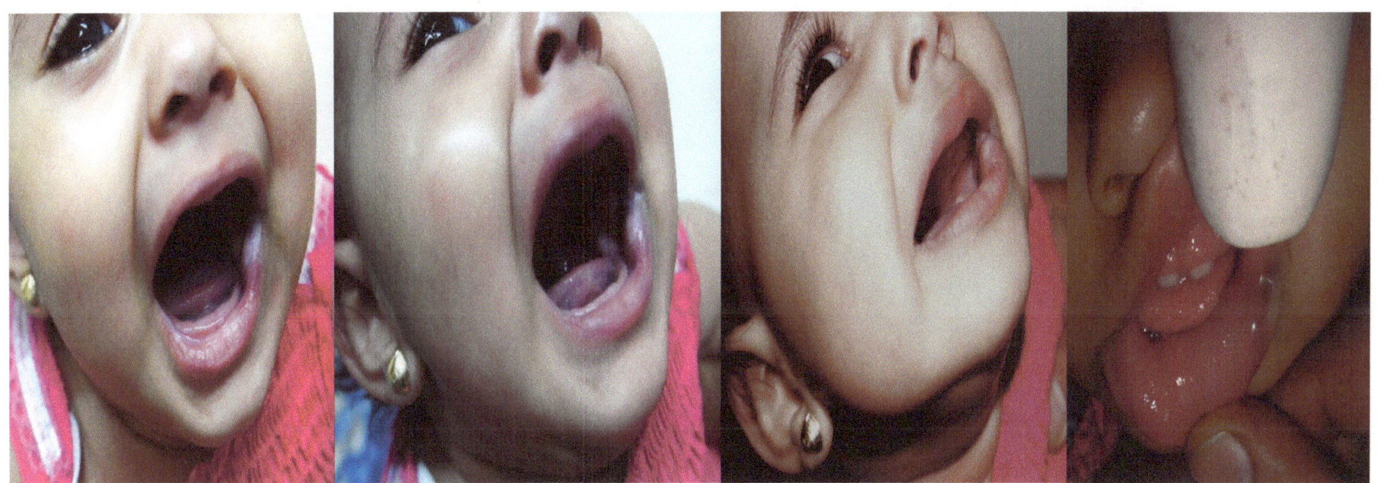

11.Inner lip resolution after 5 sessions of bleomycin injections

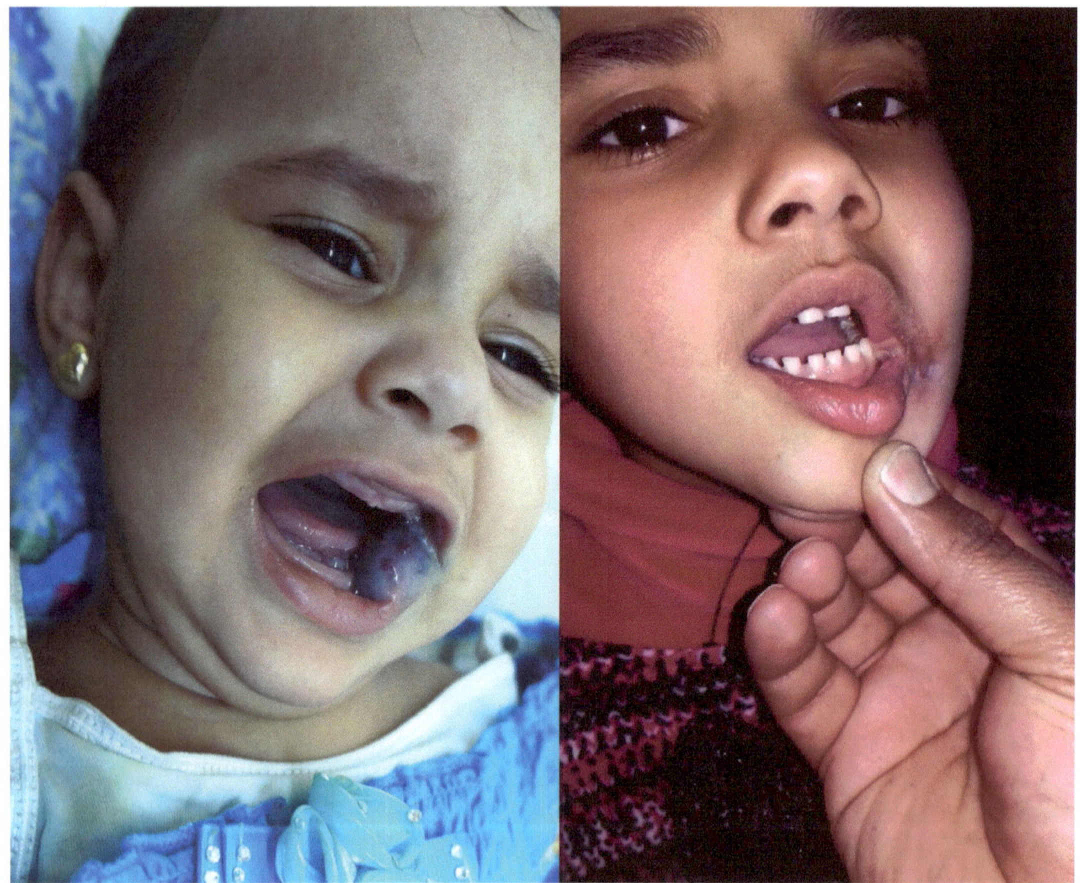

12. Local anesthetic Emla cream before bleomycin injection for a forehead hemangioma with almost complete resolution after 4 sessions of bleomycin injection for a blind girl (congenital cataract)

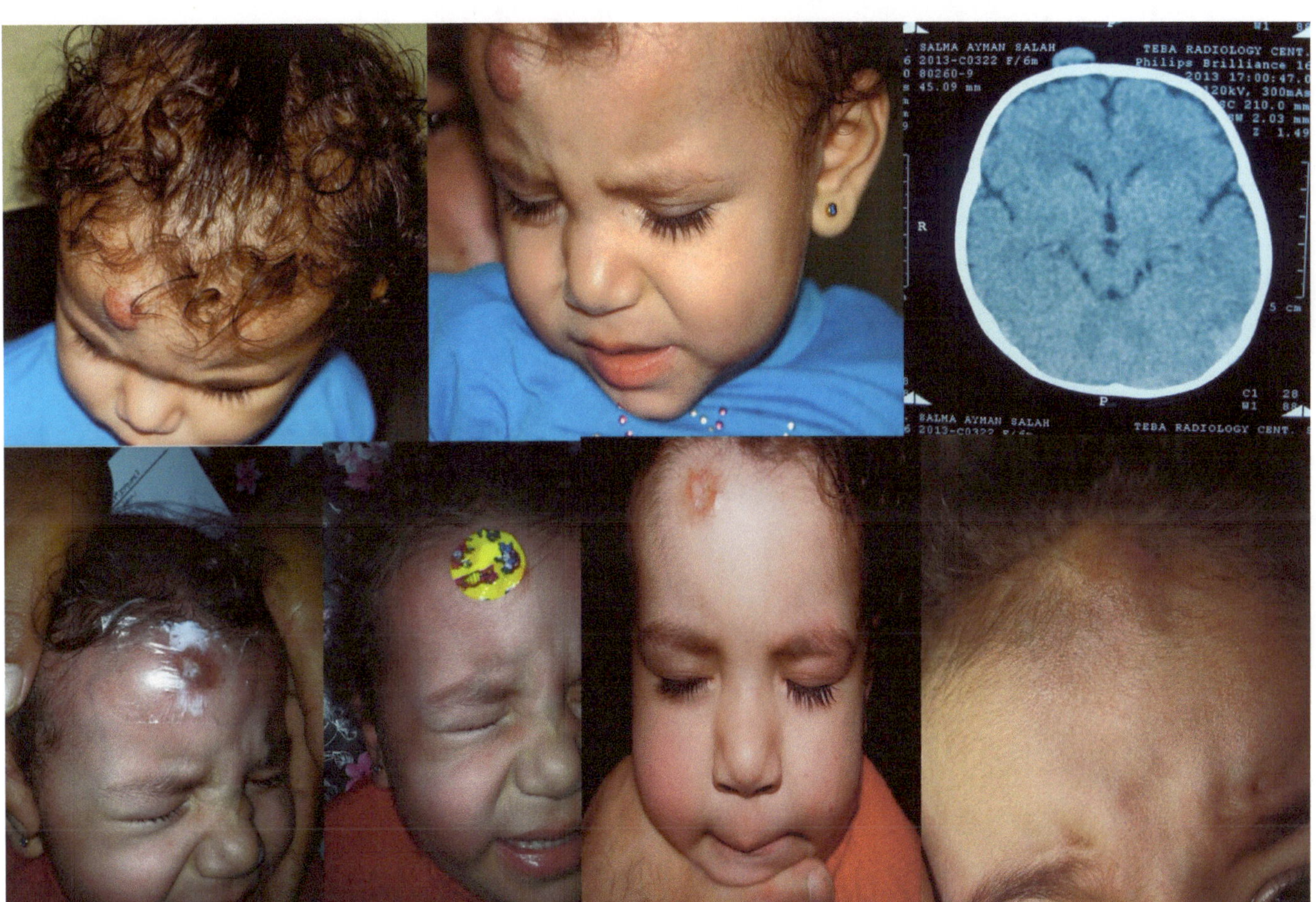

13.Small scalp hemangioma; complete resolution after 3 sessions.

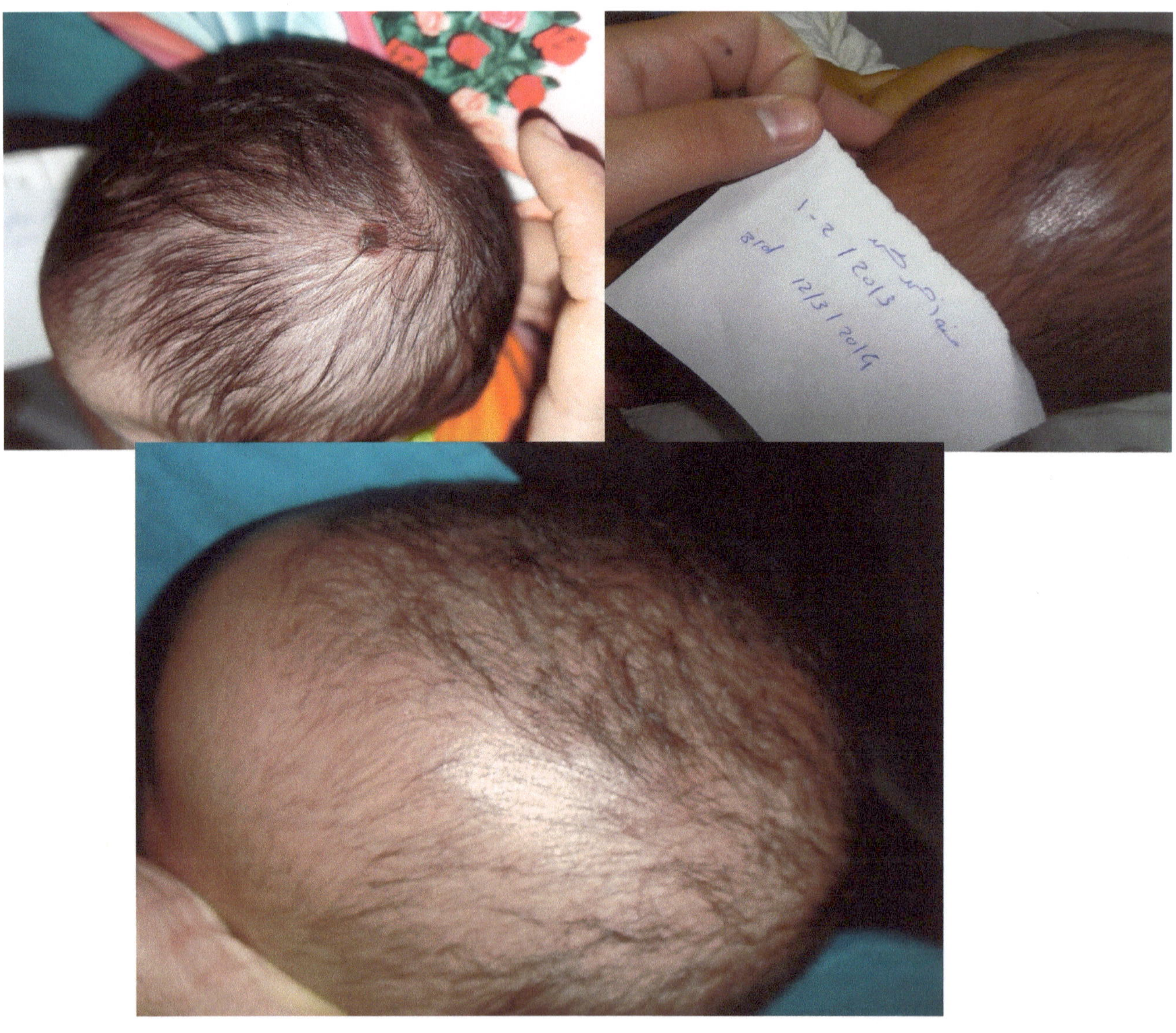

14. Combined vascular malformation (cavernous and superficial hemangioma) in the nape of the neck showed complete resolution after 4 session of bleomycin injections.

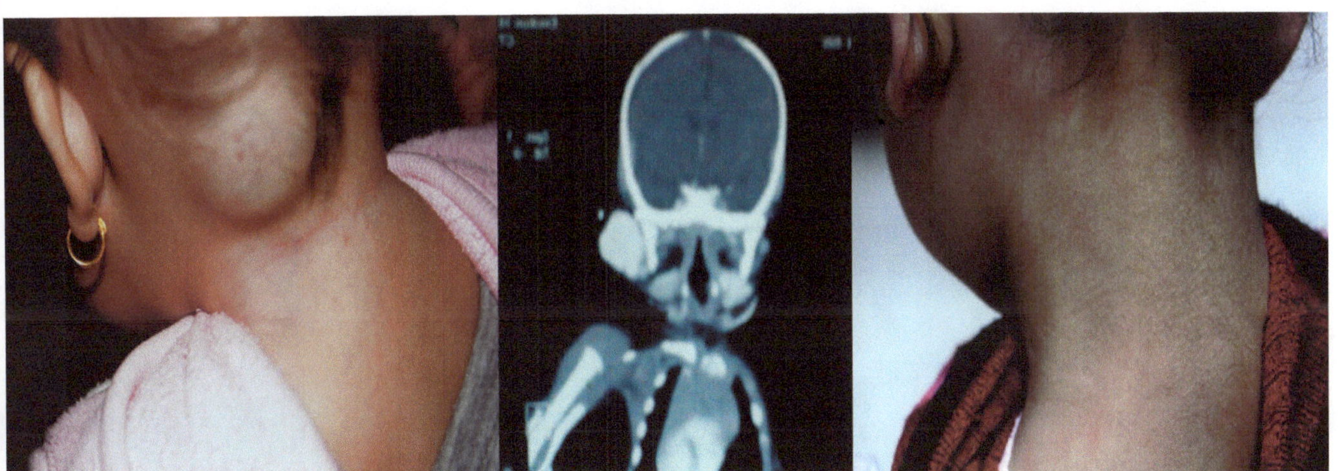

15. Nose hemangioma with complete resolution after 3 session of bleomycin injections

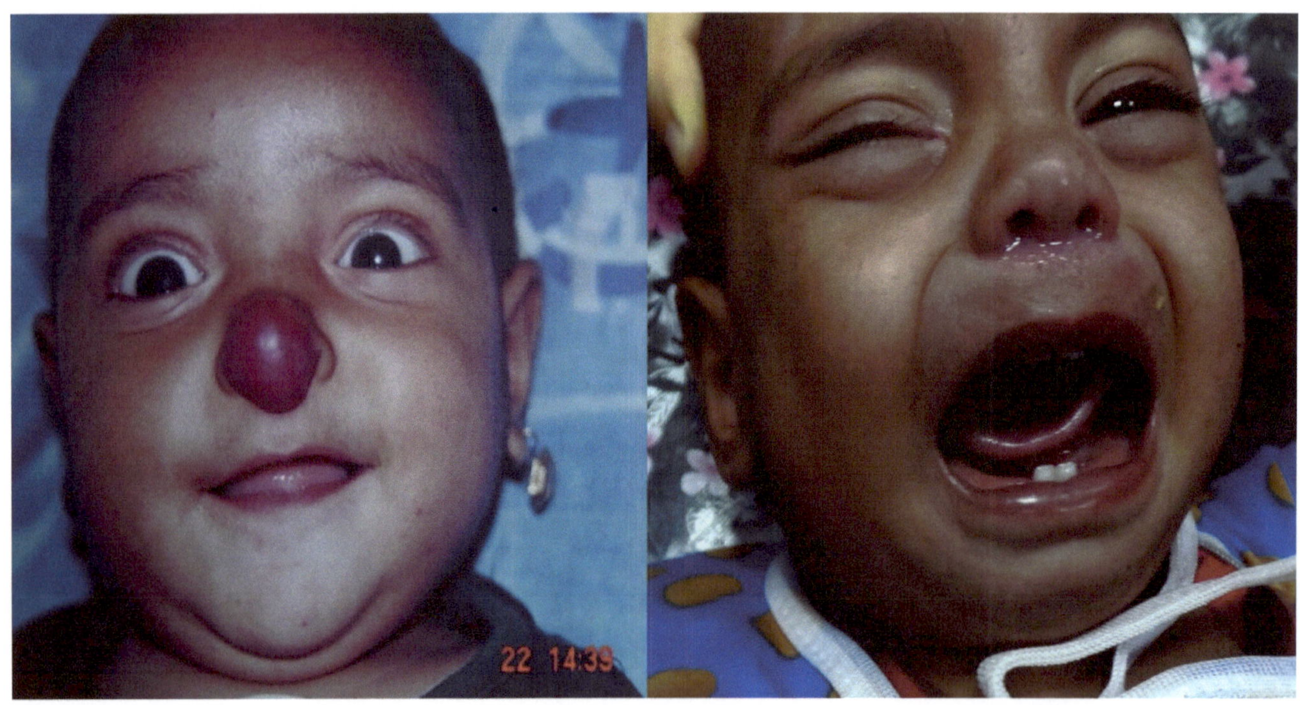

16. Superficial port-wine hemangioma showed partial response after 4 sessions of
    injection

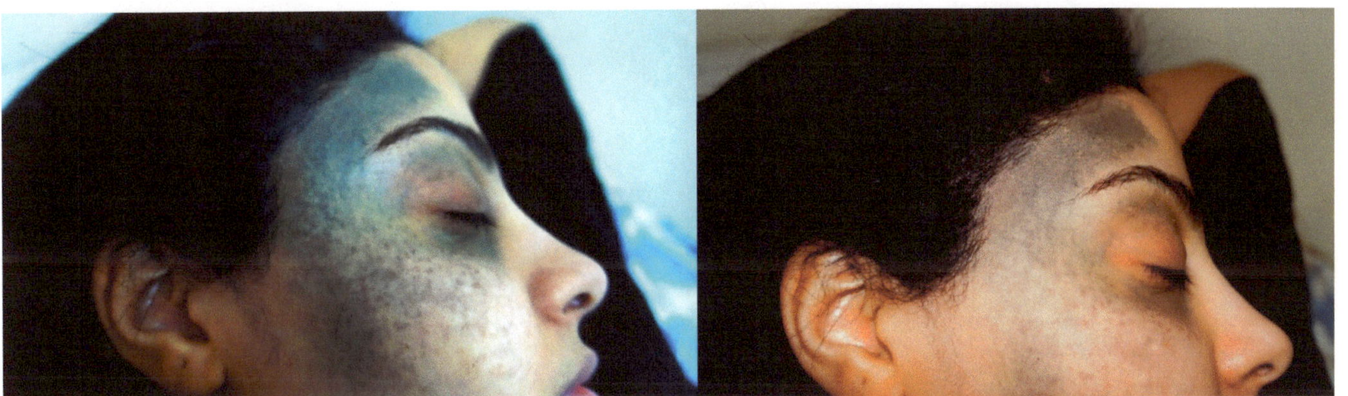

17. Severe multiple chin and chest wall hemangioma managed by 2 sessions of corticosteroid injections followed by bleomycin injections 7 sessions with partial response mainly in the chest wall

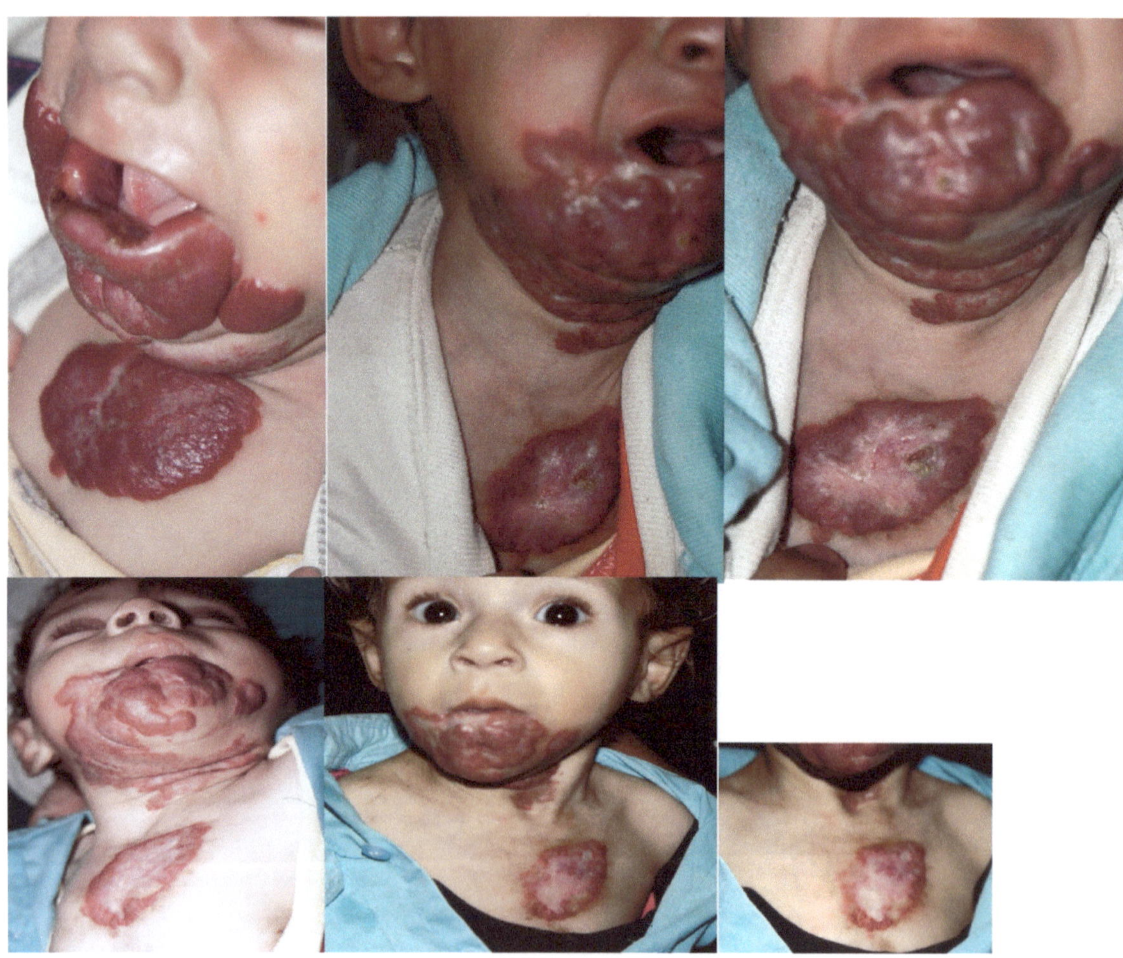

18.Chest wall hemangioma with 80% response after 3 sessions, but complicated

with a superficial ulceration.

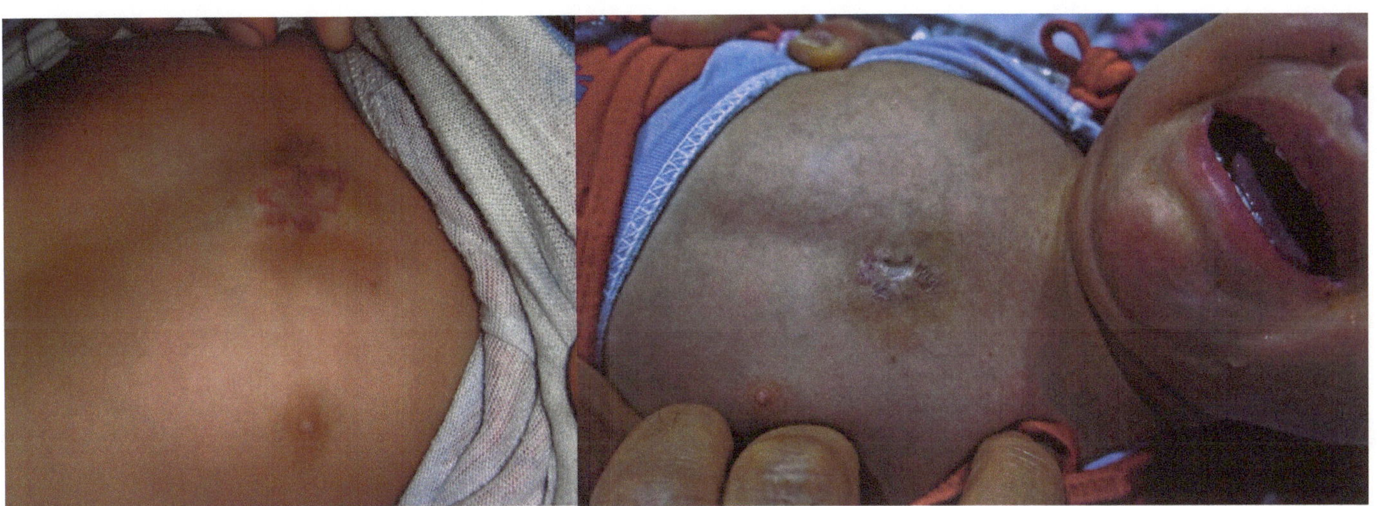

19. Labial hemangioma in 2 years old girl; showed complete resolution after 4 sessions of bleomycin injection

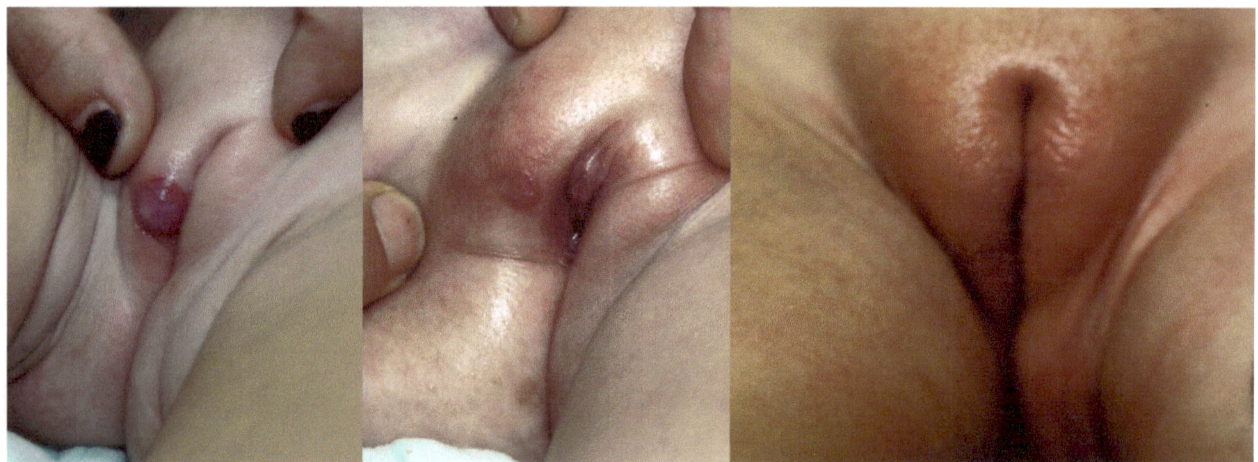

20. Extensive anal hemangioma in a neonate resolved completely after 5sessions
   of bleomycin injection

25

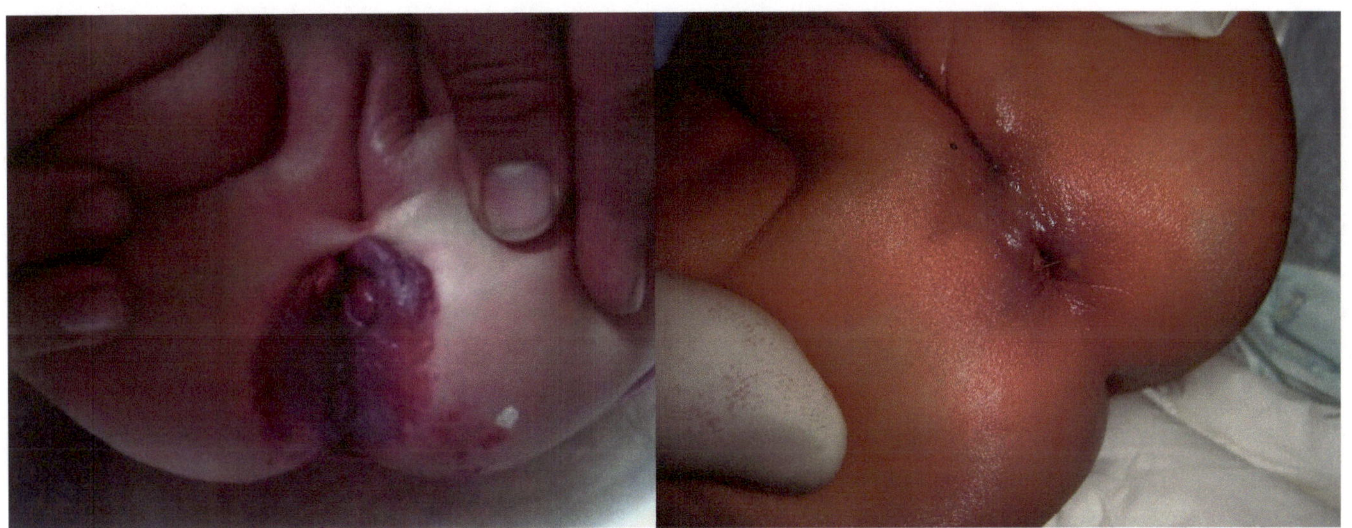

21.Cavernous anal hemangioma resolved completely after 2 sessions of corticosteroid injections followed by 4 sessions of bleomycin injection

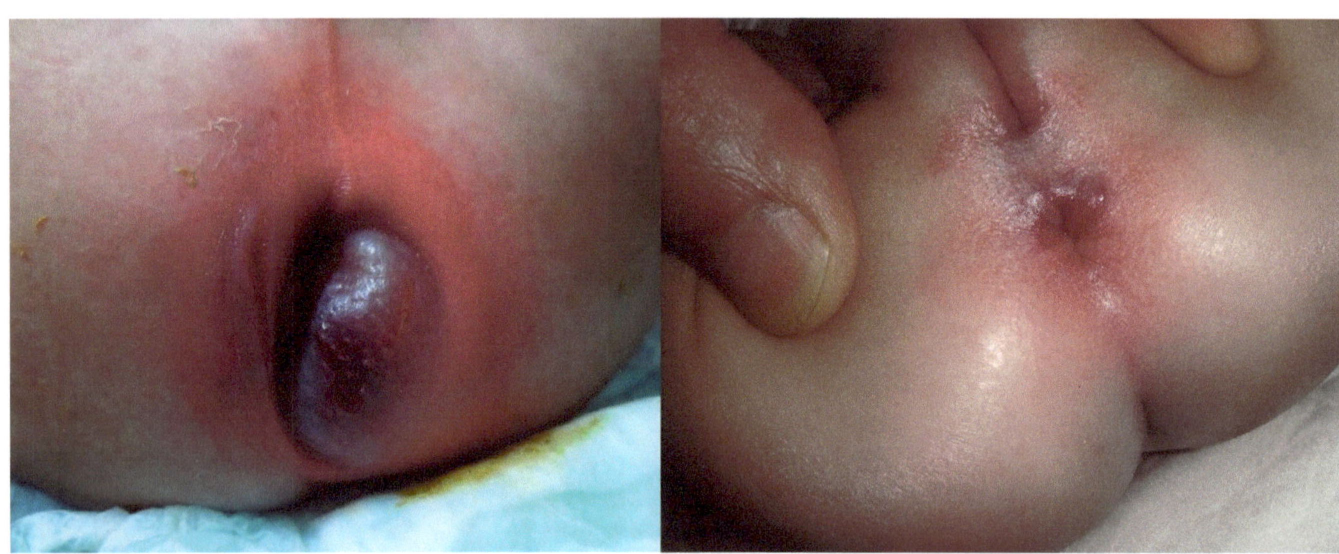

22. Different complications of bleomycin injection for hemangioma:

- Upper lip remnant scar
- Lower lip tissue loss
- Chest wall necrosis
- Forehead ulceration
- Chest wall infection and necrosis
- Hypodermic scar of forearm
- Minimal infection
- Chin infection
- Cavernous hemangioma of the knee; failure to respond and superficial necrosis

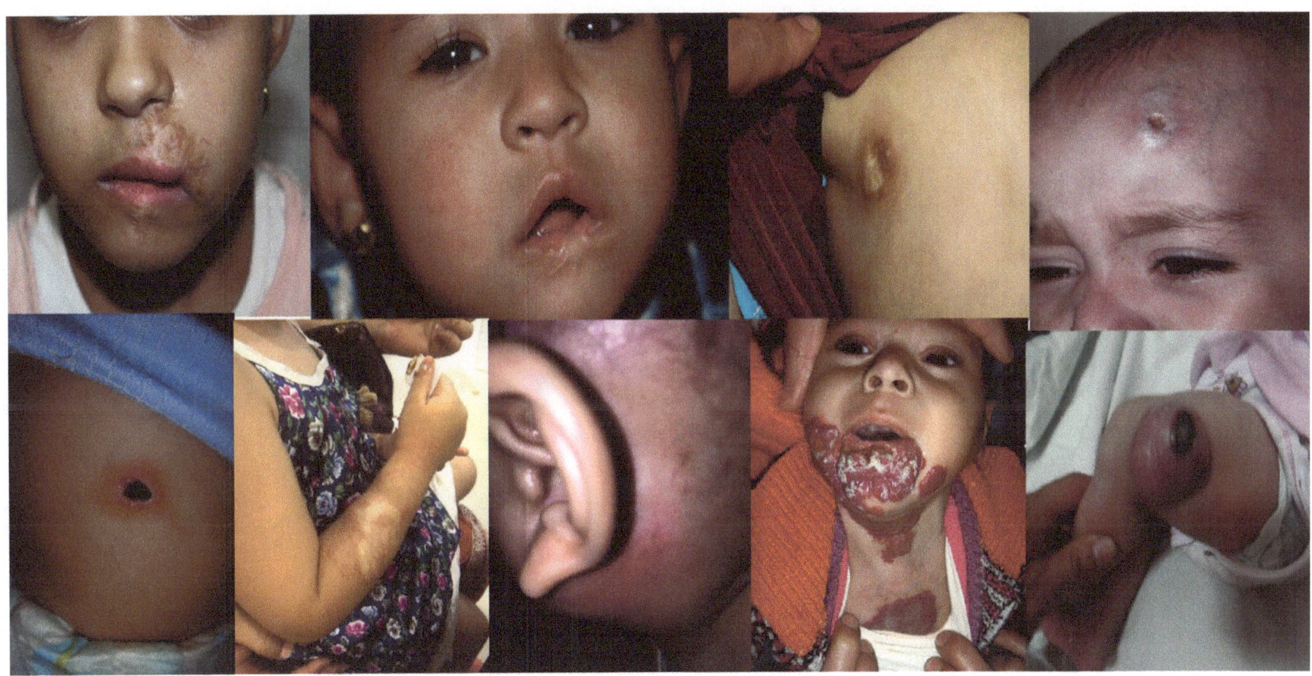

23. Cheek hemangioma excised surgically, after failure to respond to 3 sessions of bleomycin injection.

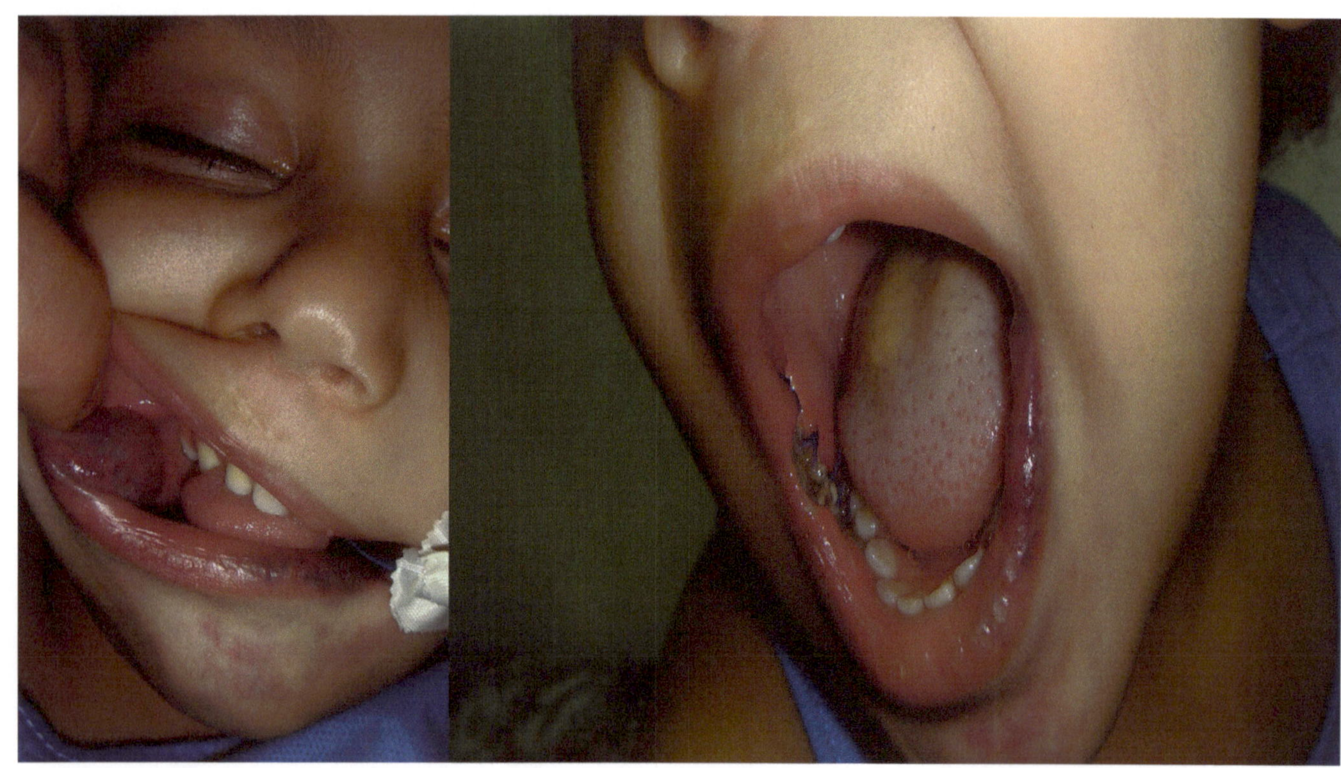

24.Forehead failed to respond to bleomycin excised surgically

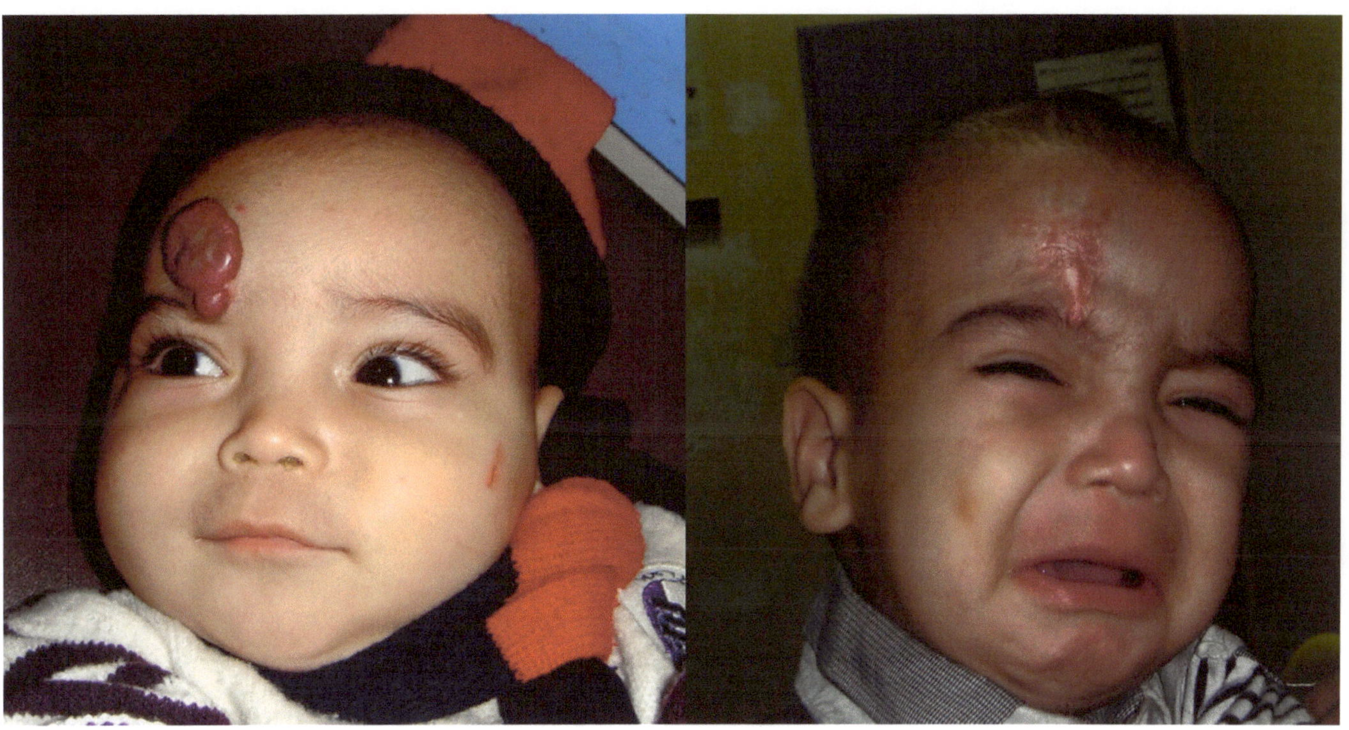

25.Cavernous huge hemangioma of the abdominal wall excised surgically

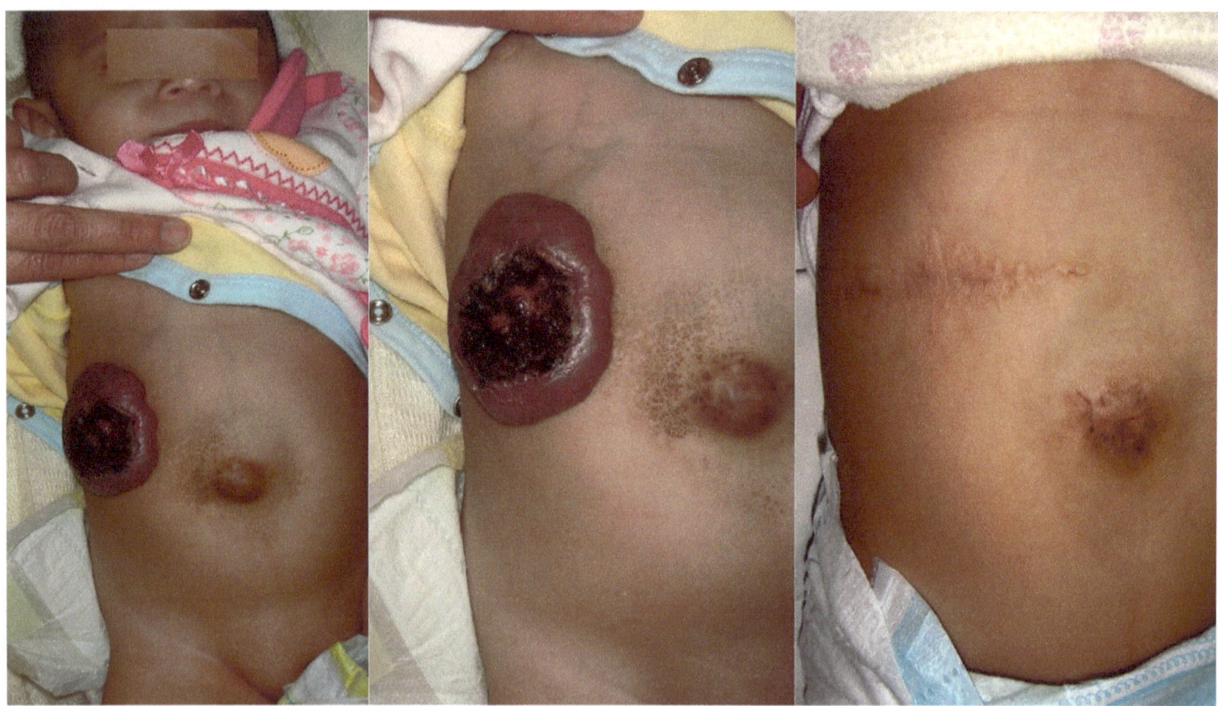

26.Forehead hemangioma excised surgically after failure to respond to bleomycin

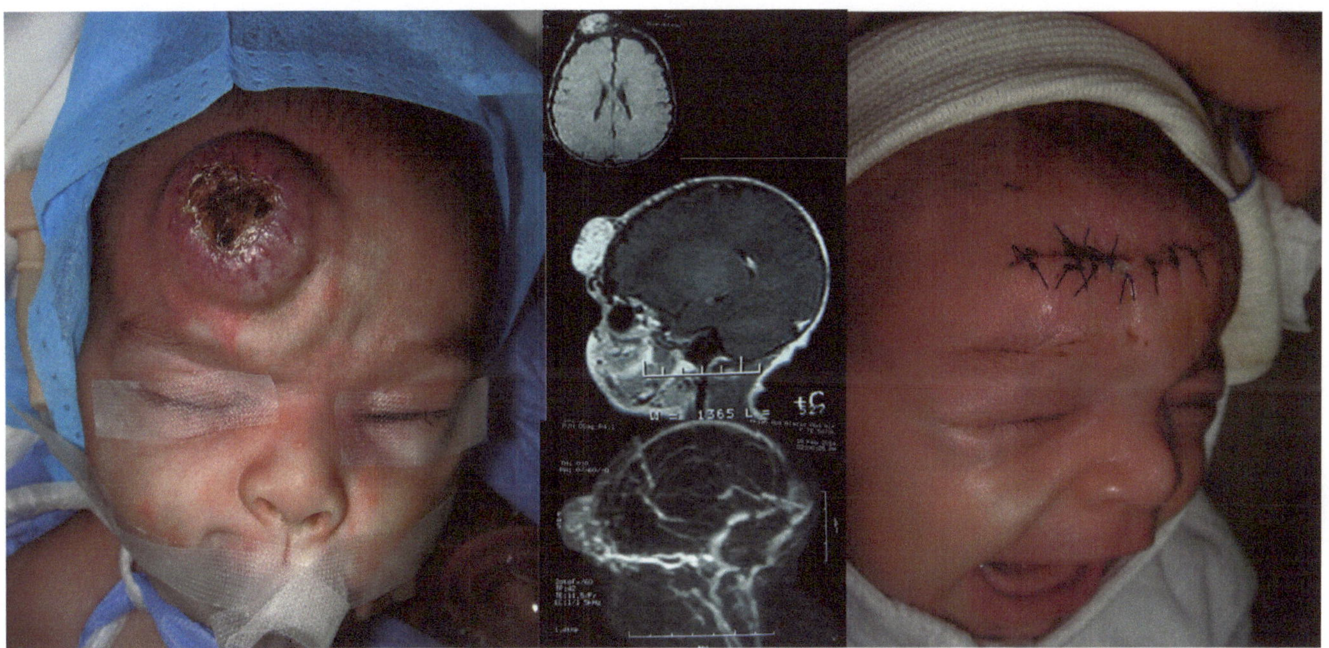

27.Z-plasty and excision of a neck hemangioma

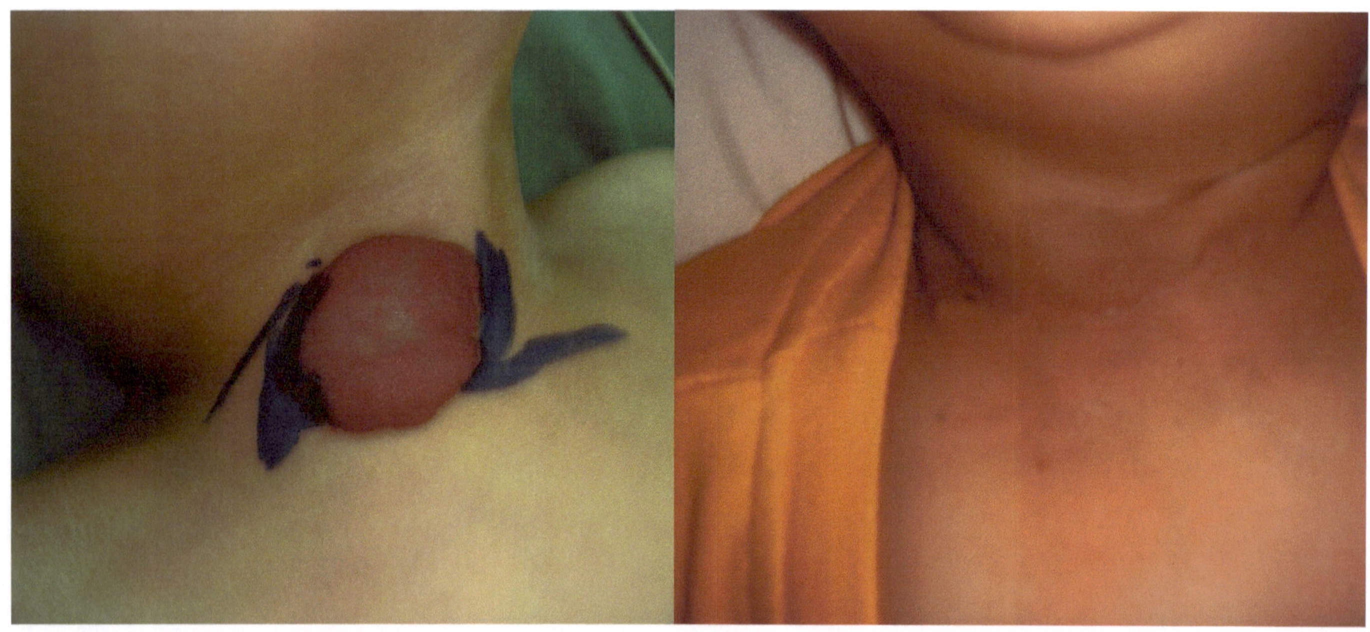

28.Shoulder hemangioma excised

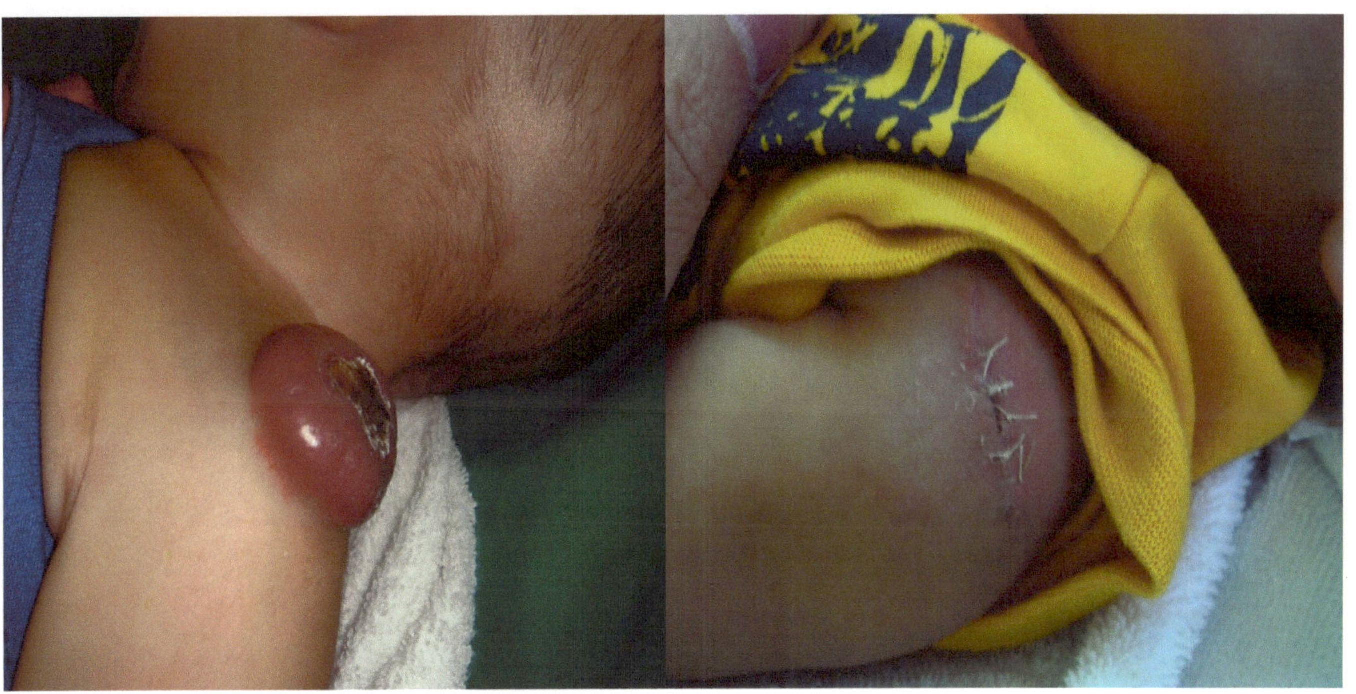

29.Superficial abdominal wall hemangioma managed by two stages of tissue expansion and excision.

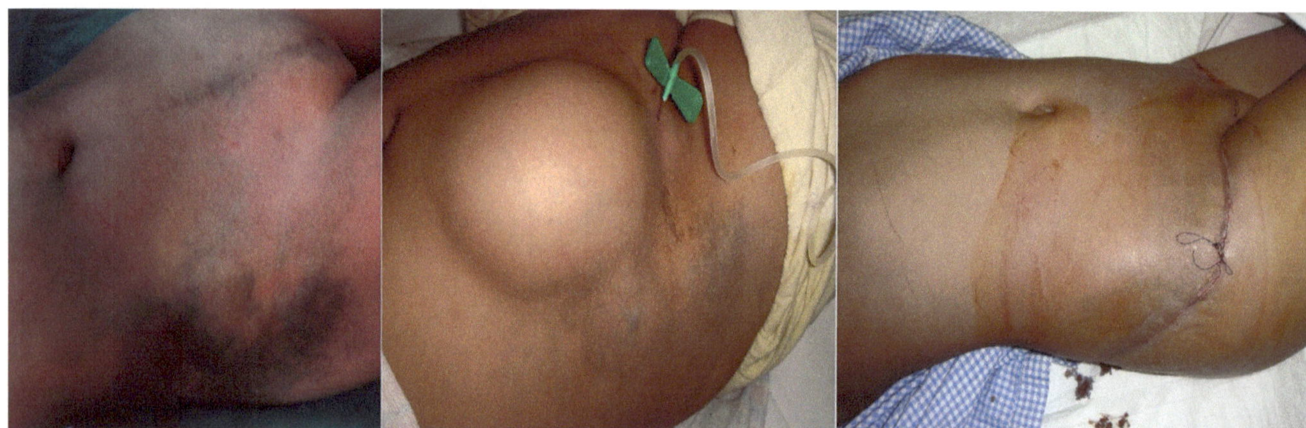

30. Abdominal wall large cavernous hemangioma managed by tissue expansion
and surgical excision.

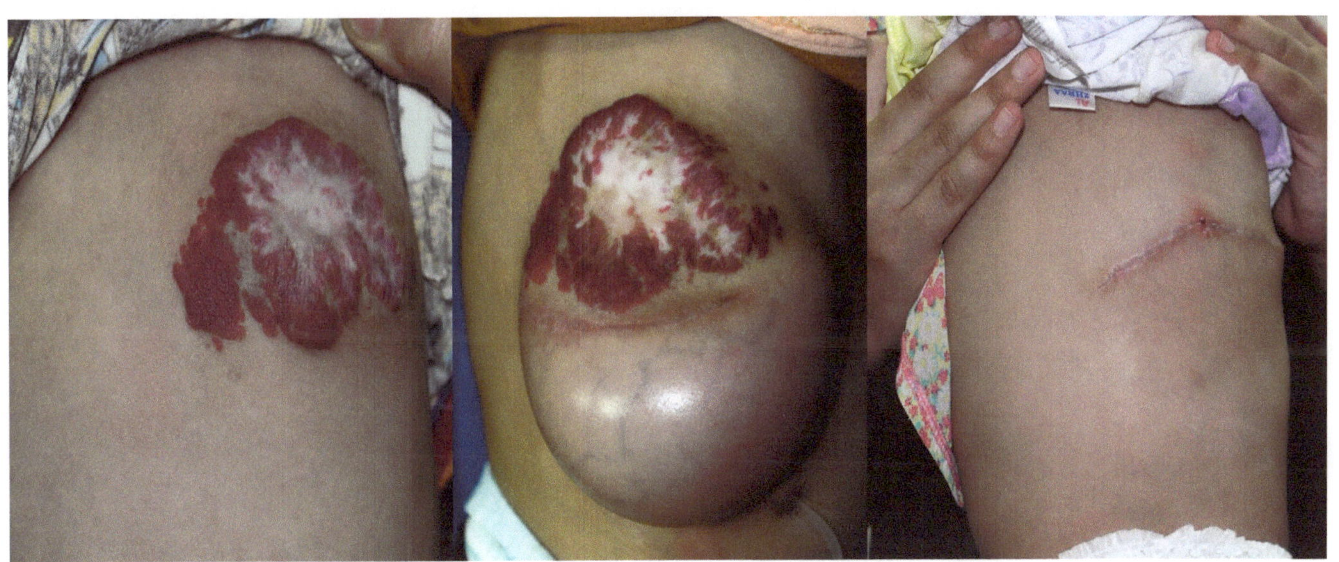

31.Extensive ulcerated hemangioma of the face and scalp managed by sequential bleomycin injections, tissue expansion and excision eventually.

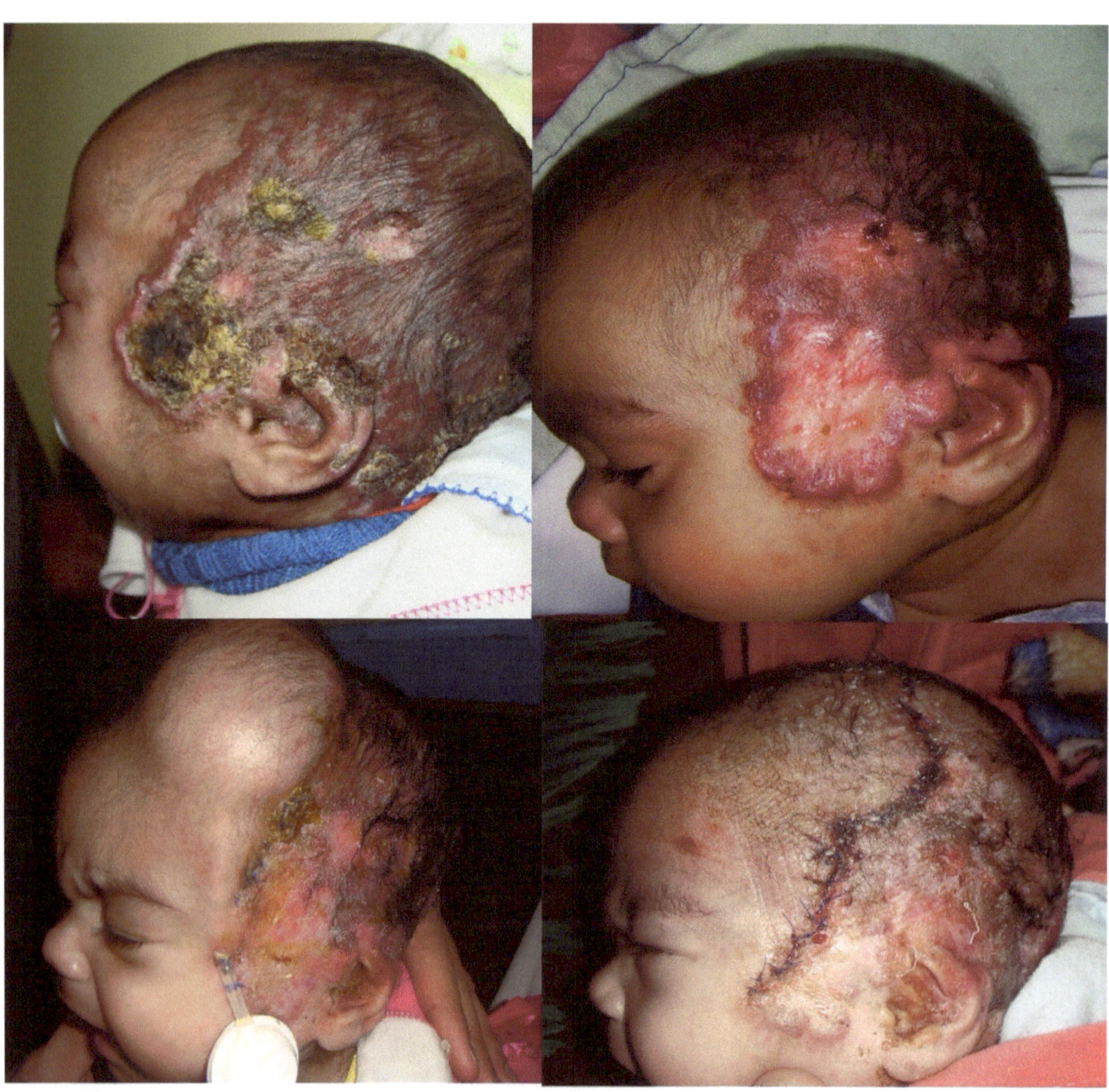

32. Extensive penile, scrotal and suprapubic hemangioma and vascular
   malformation managed from the age of 6 months up to the age of 12 years with
   bleomycin injections, tissue expansion, excision and remedy for 12 sessions
   along 10 years, with a reasonable outcome.

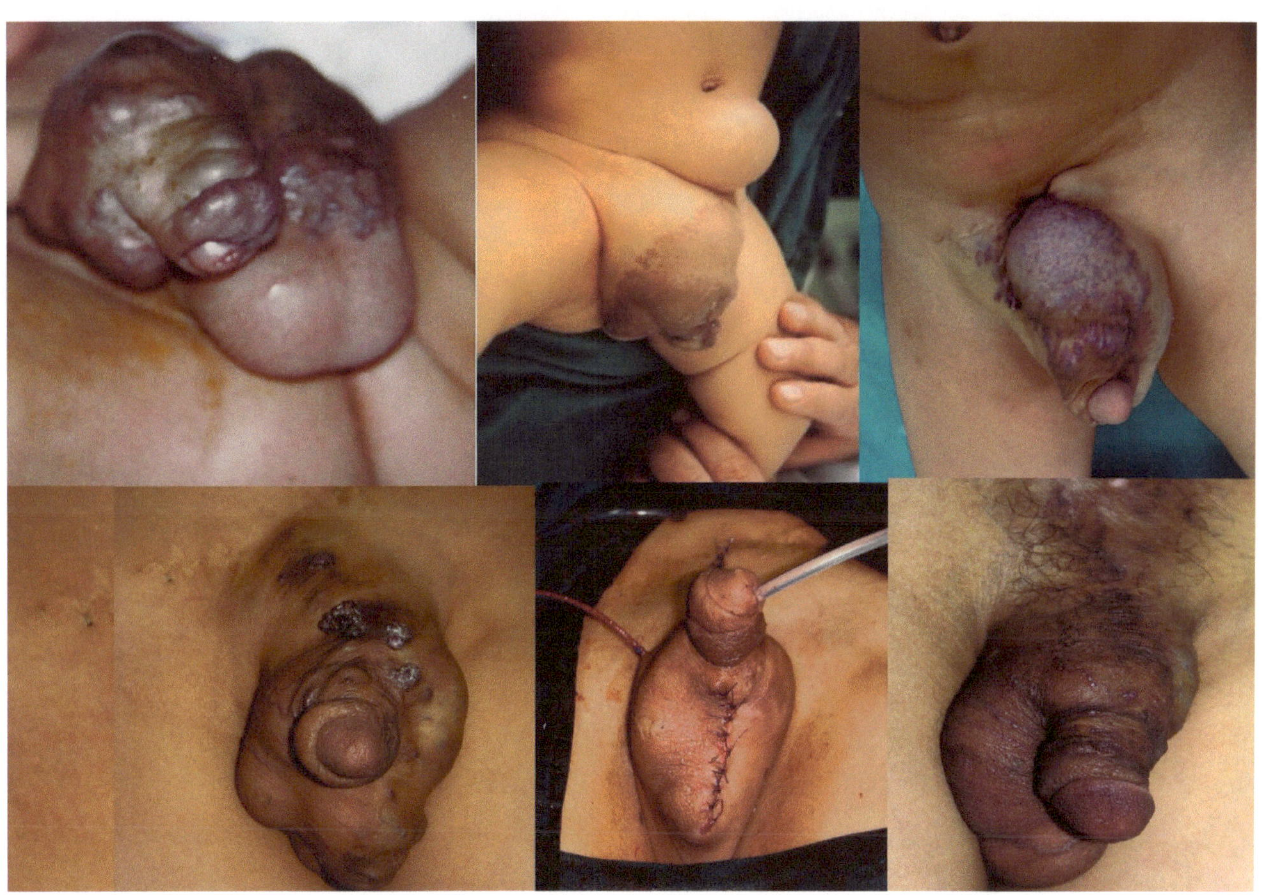

33. The same previous patient with bleomycin injection for a residual hemangioma
at the age of 20 years.

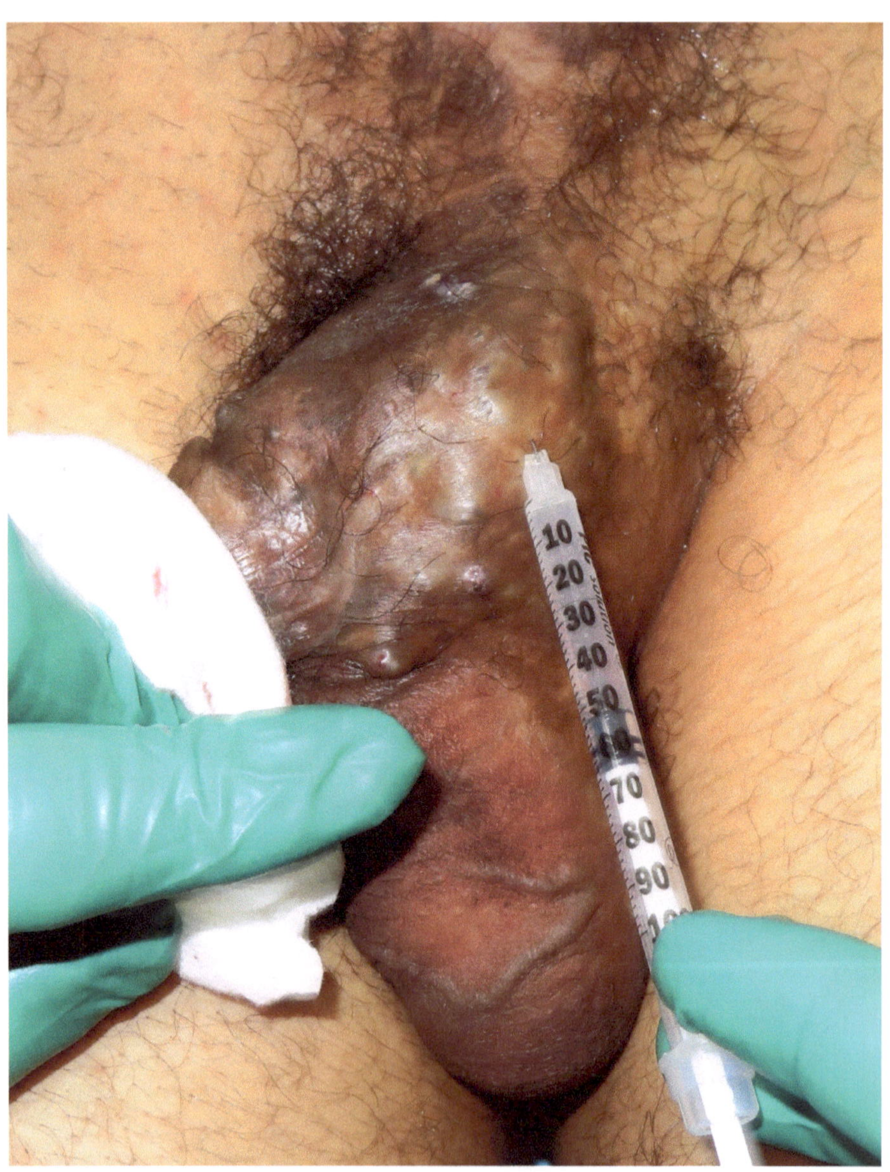

34., a, b Different presentations of lymphatic malformations:

- Combined lymphatic and hygrometers axillary malformation
- Combined lymphangioma an hemangioma in the supraclavicular region
- Hourglass cystic hygroma affecting both the axilla and root of the neck
- Huge chin, submandibular and parotid cystic hygroma
- Rarely; the lymphatic malformations may affect the thigh
- Sublingual cystic hygroma resembling Ranula
- Breast cystic hygroma
- Antenatally detected neck cystic hygroma managed through EXIT

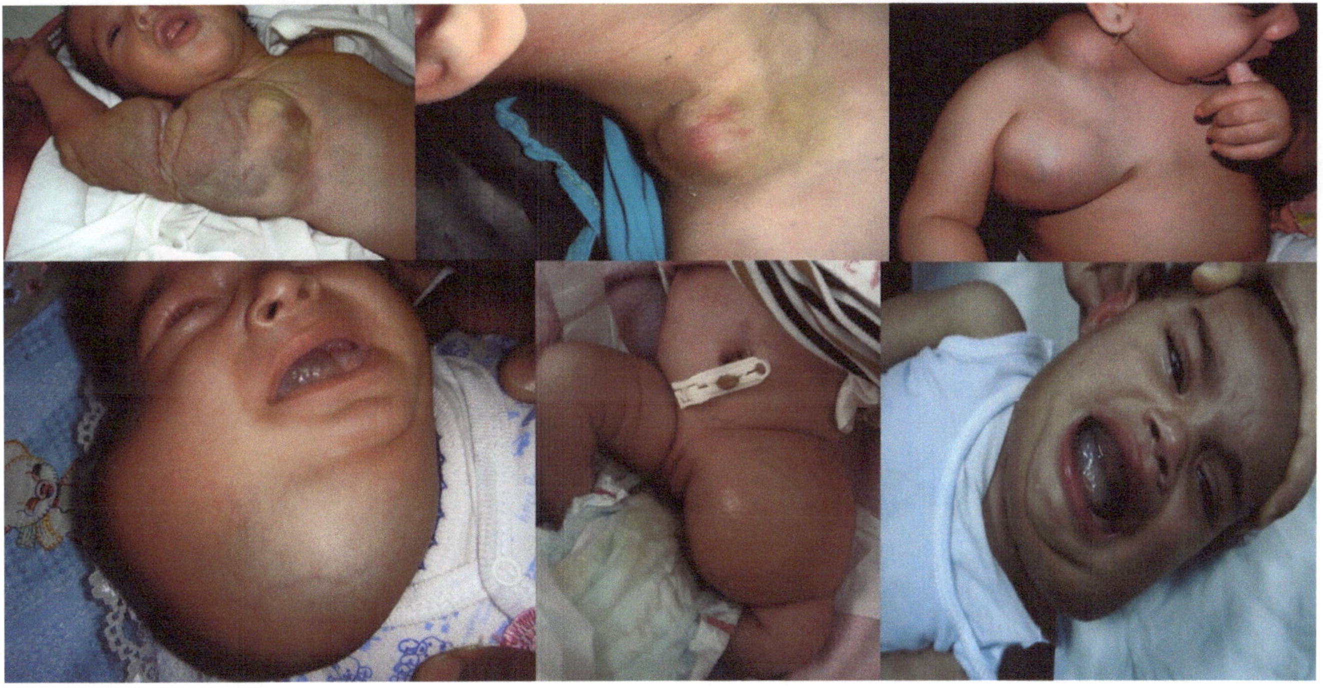

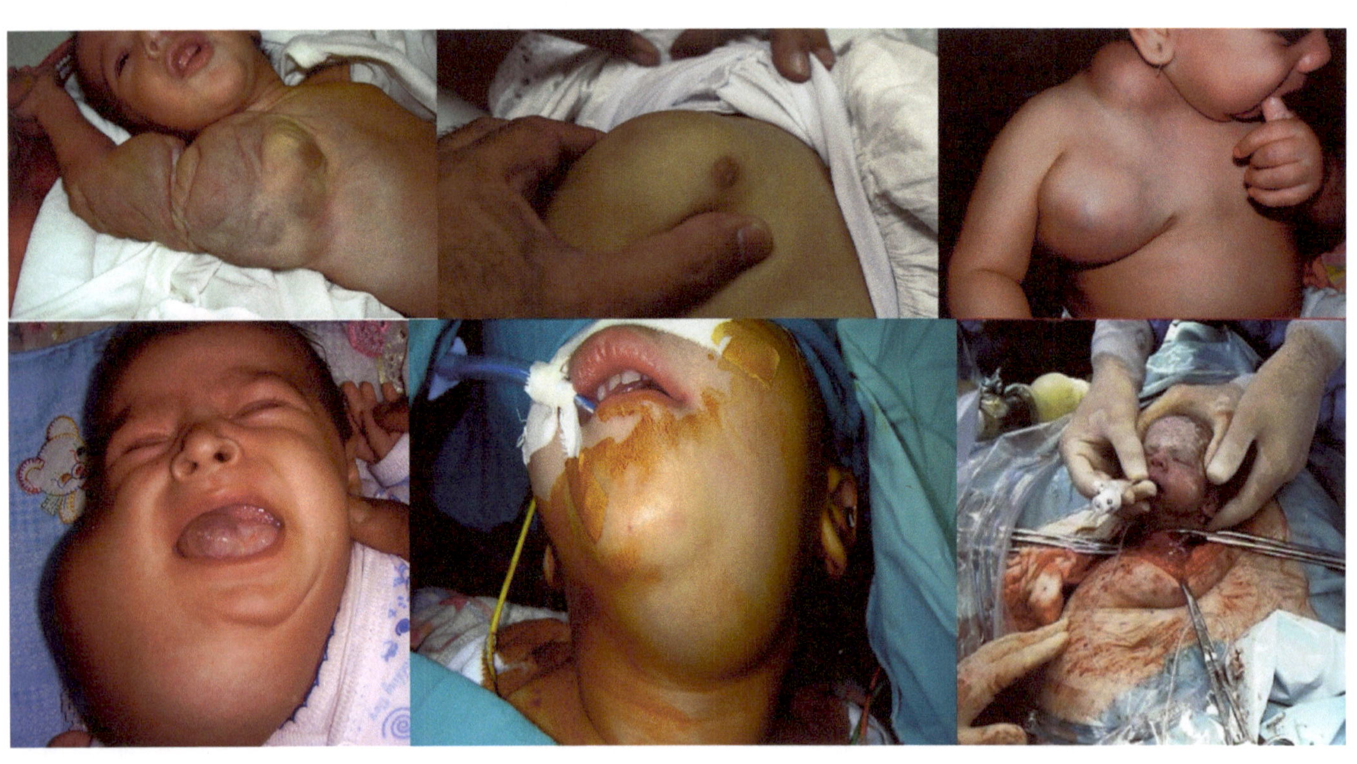

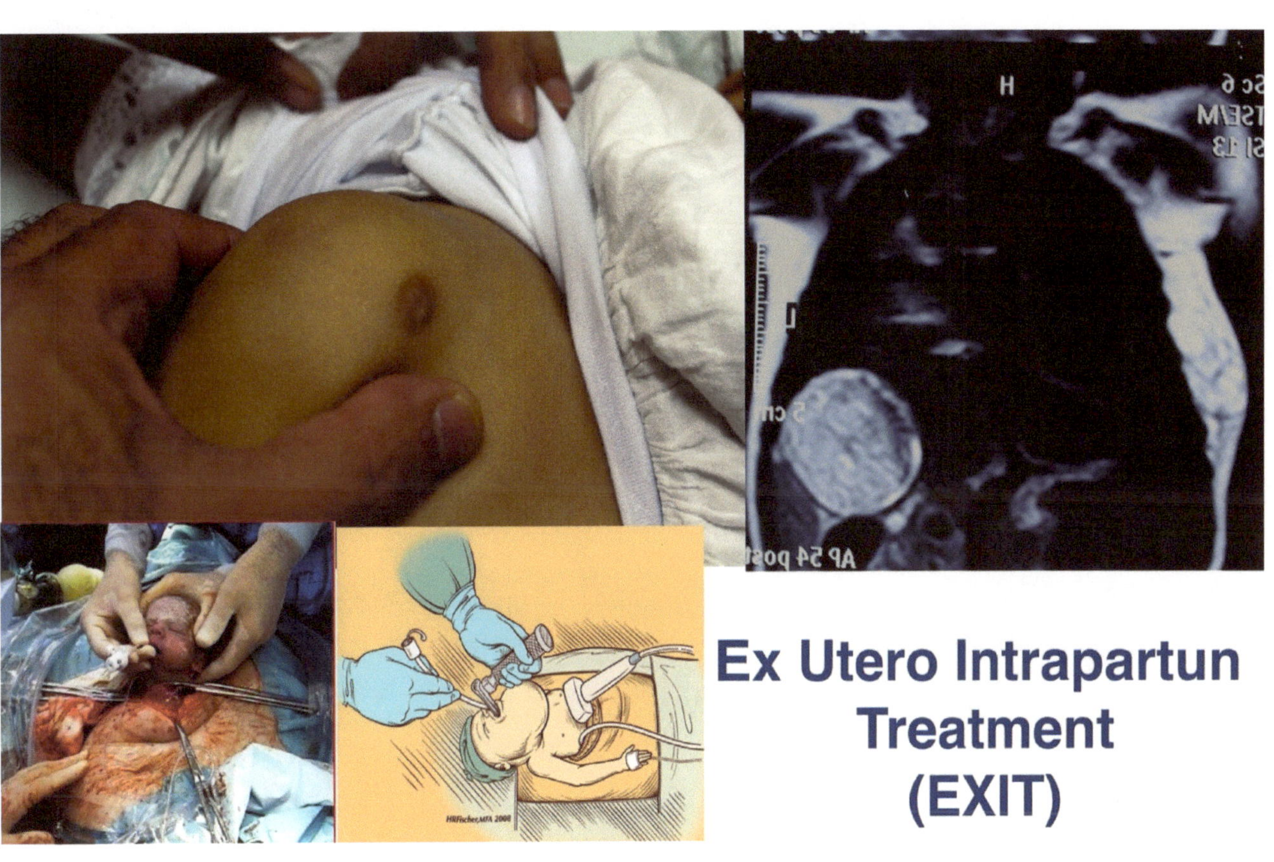

Ex Utero Intrapartun Treatment (EXIT)

Different Modalities of Bleomycin injections

Different Modalities of Bleomycin injections

Our protocol for bleomycin injection for hemangioma and LMs is to use this drug through one of those three ways:

- Direct injection for hemangioma followed by compression
- Aspiration of the lymphatic fluid and compensating bleomycin injection for cystic hygroma through a three-way connection
- Seeding of the resection bed after excision to avoid recurrence

35.Different modalities of bleomycin injection for LMs; either direct injection,

dual aspiration preceding injection or injection of the surgical bed to avoid

recurrence

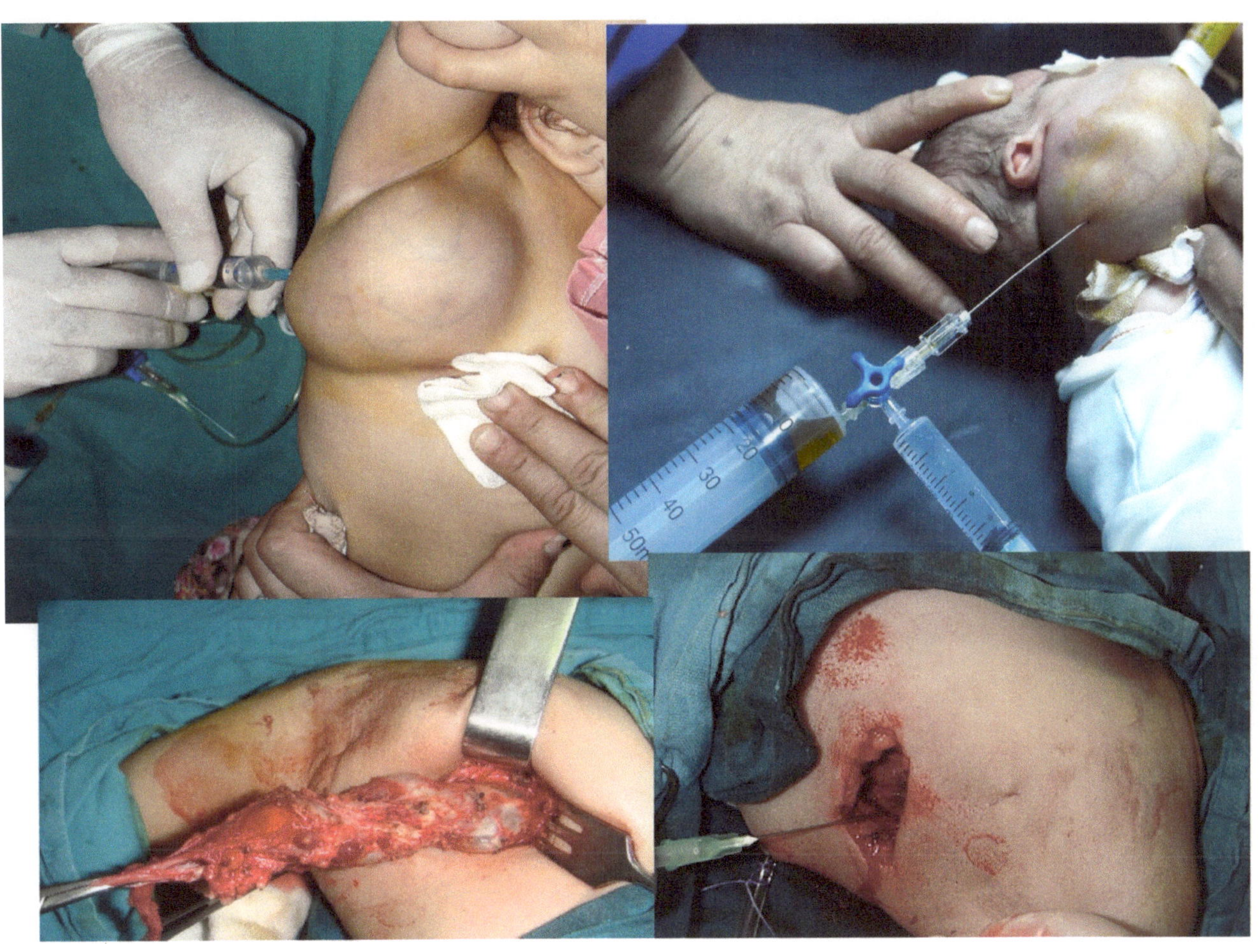

36.Small axillary cystic hygroma resolved completely after 2 sessions of injection

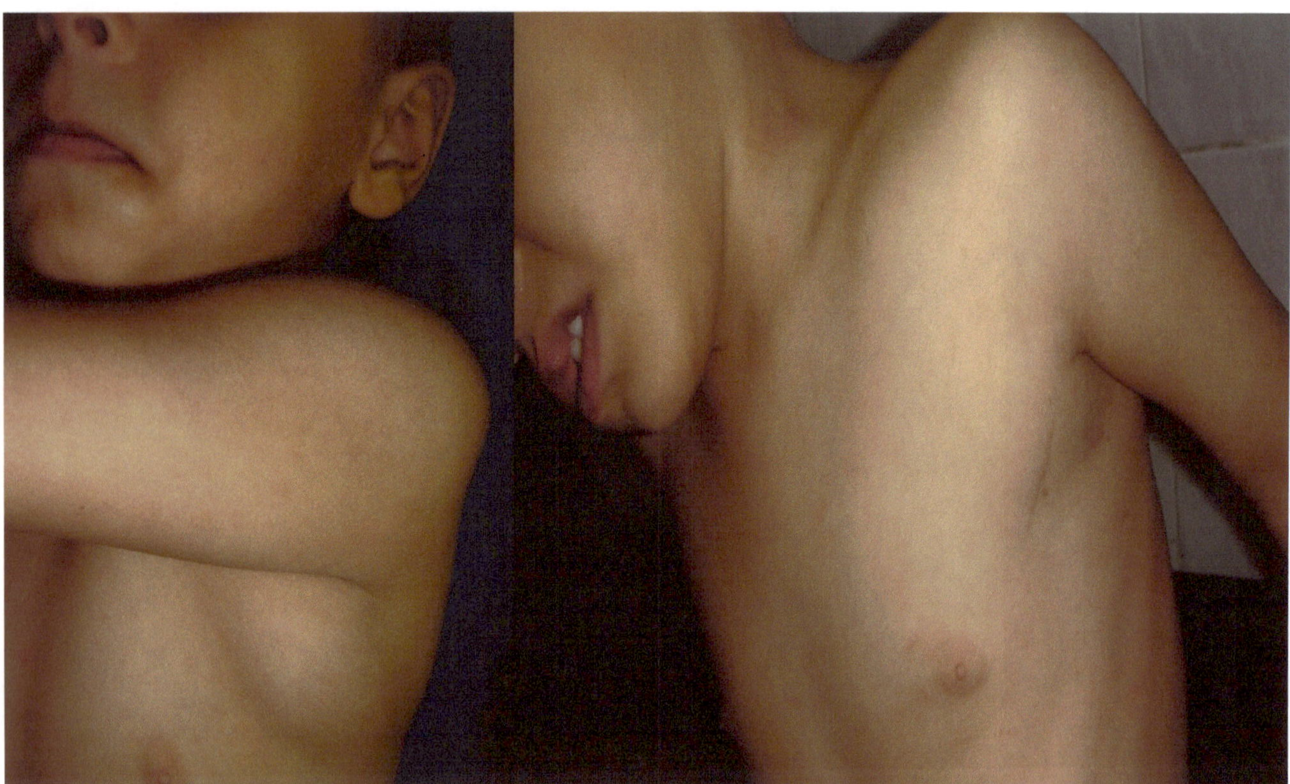

37.Huge neck cystic hygroma injected after aspiration for 6 sessions and 4 years follow up with a minimal residual injected again.

45

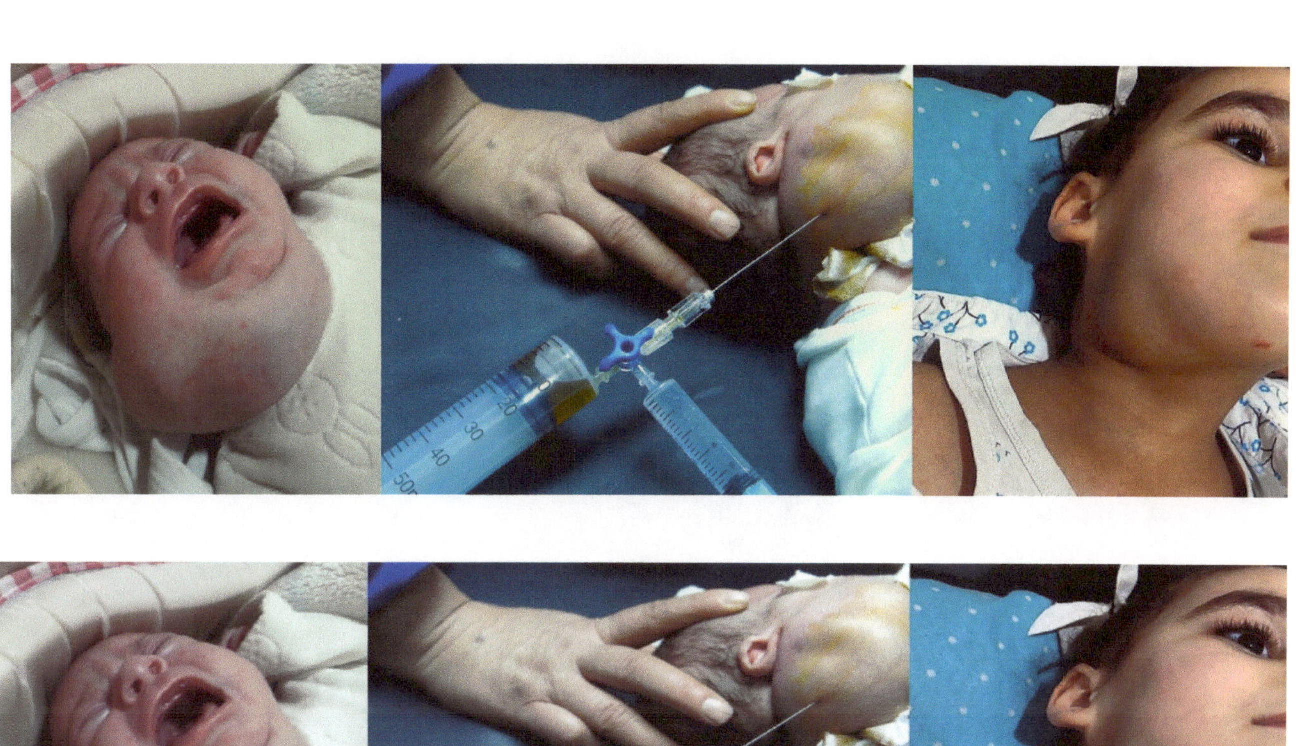

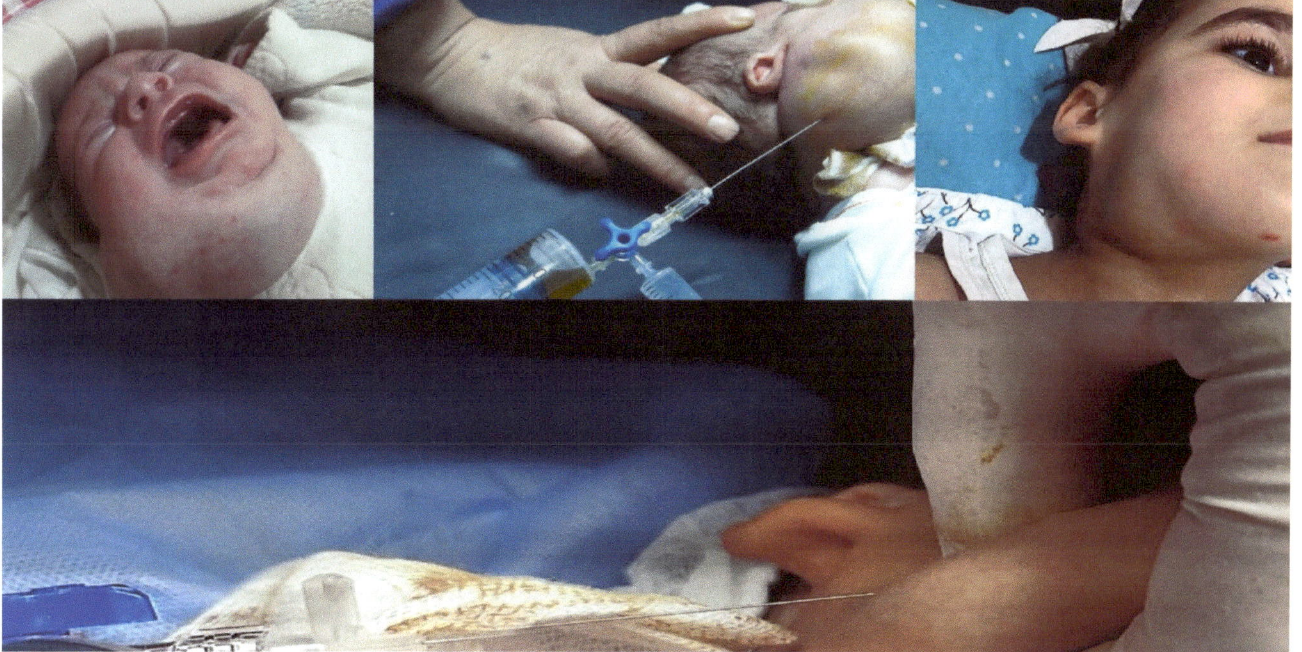

38.The same patient developed a secondary axillary hygroma at the age of 2 years

46

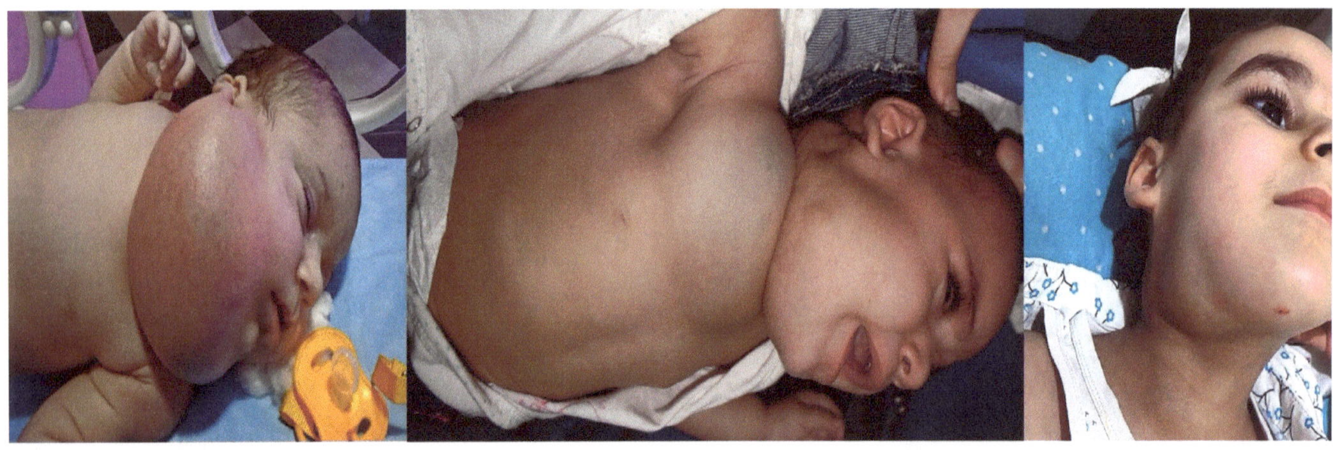

39. The sequences of the same patient with a MRI showing residual
lymphangioma at the age of 5 years, which was recently injected.

47

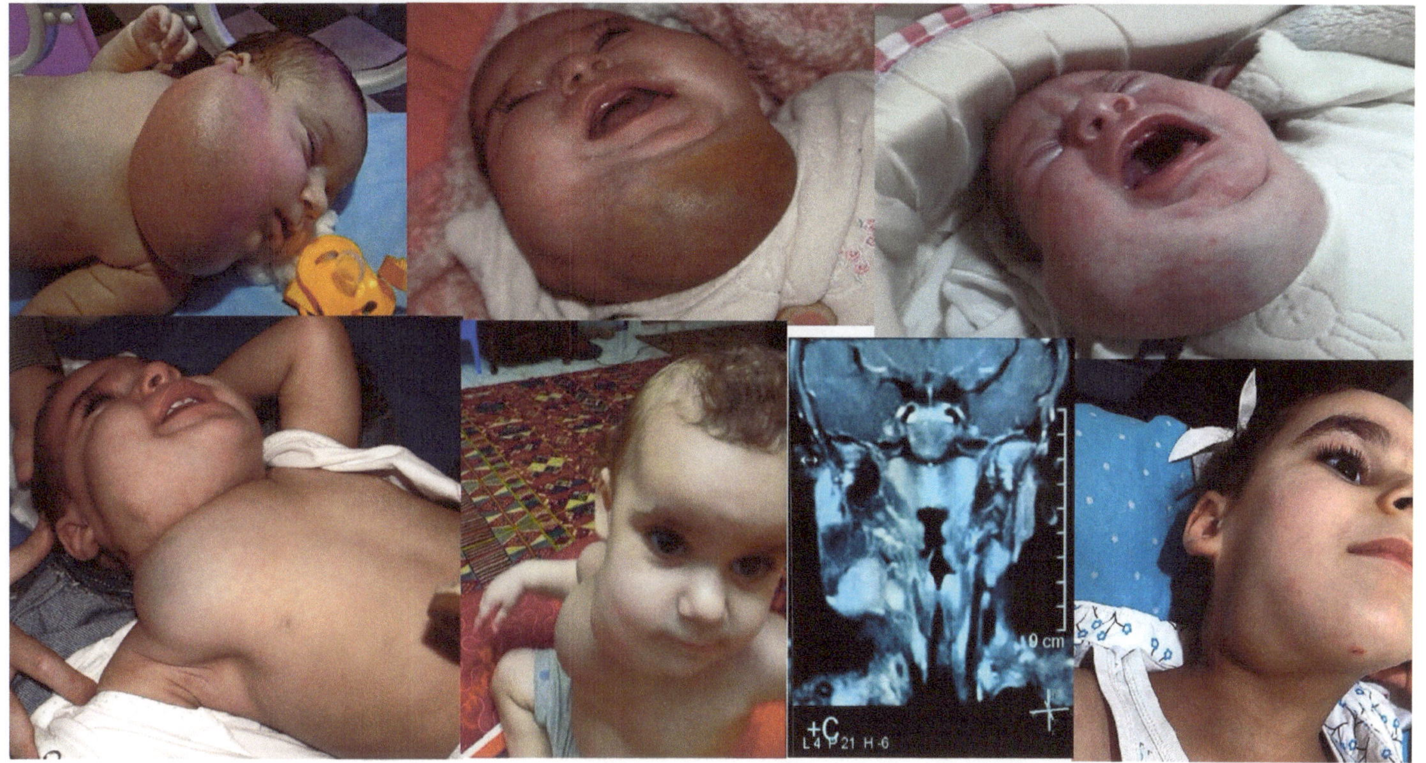

40.Localised cystic hygroma in the nape of the neck resolved completely after 2 session of bleomycin injection

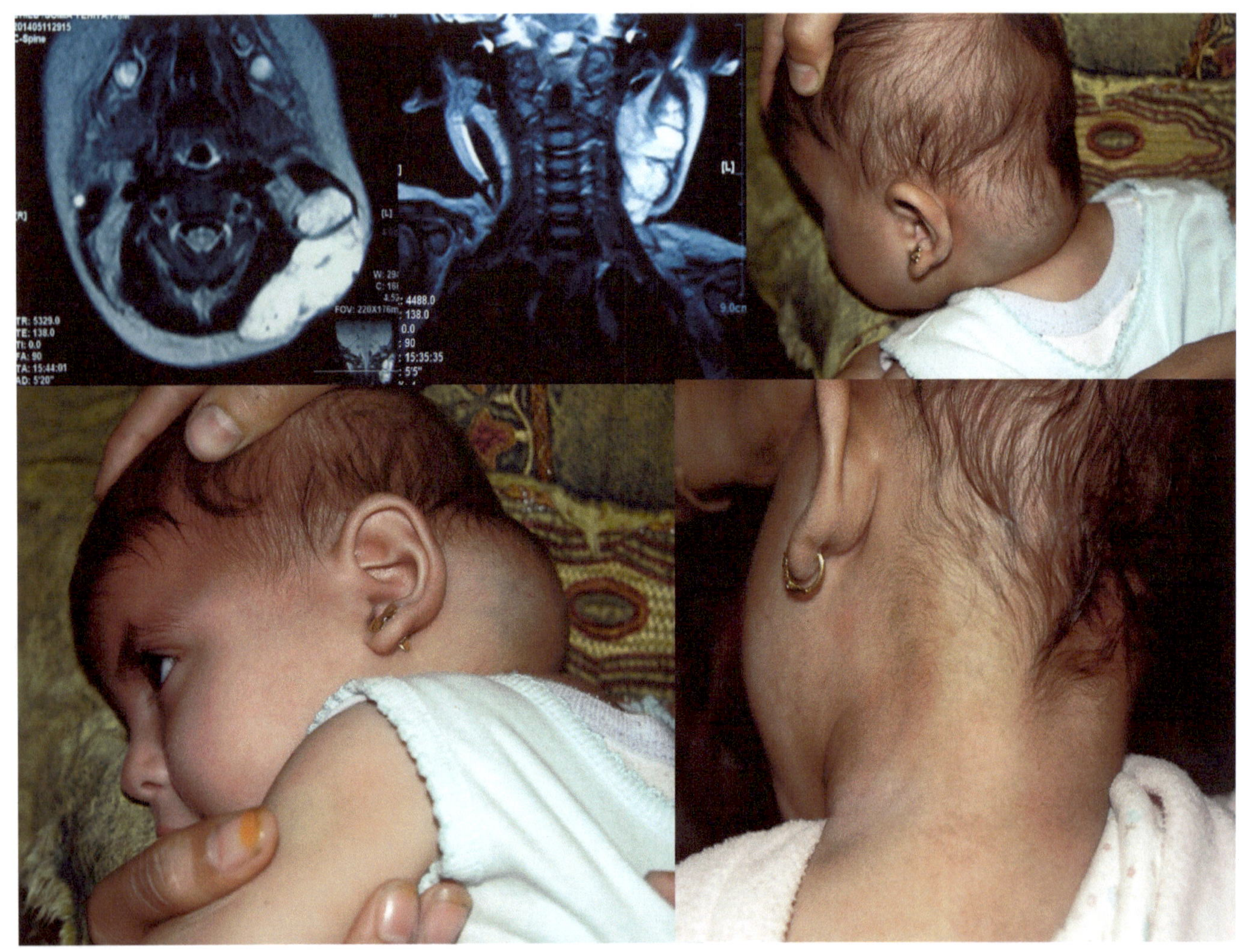

48

41.Tongue cystic hygroma resolved after 4 sessions of injection

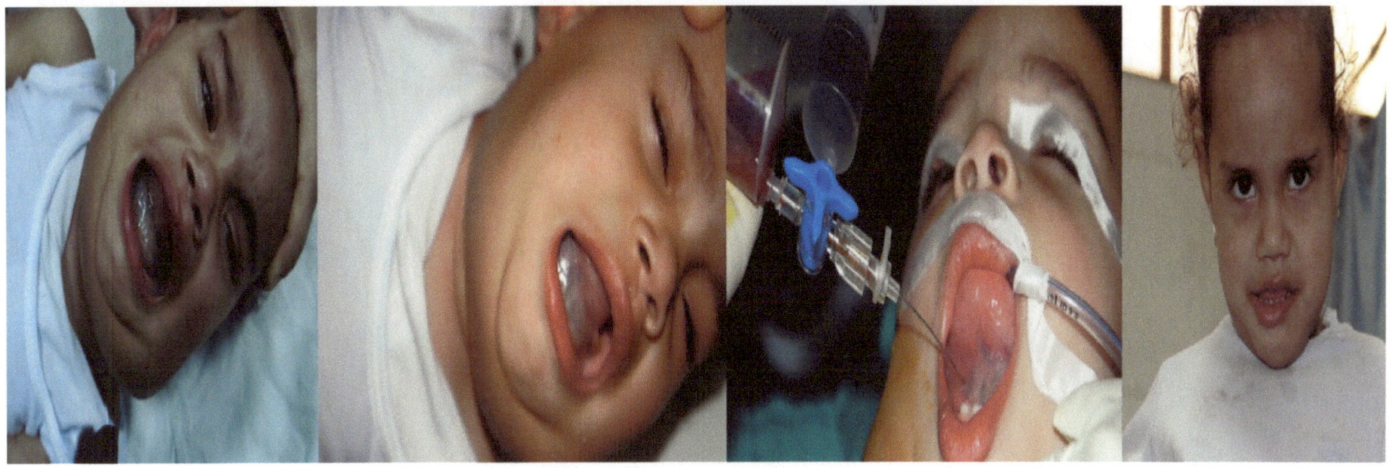

50

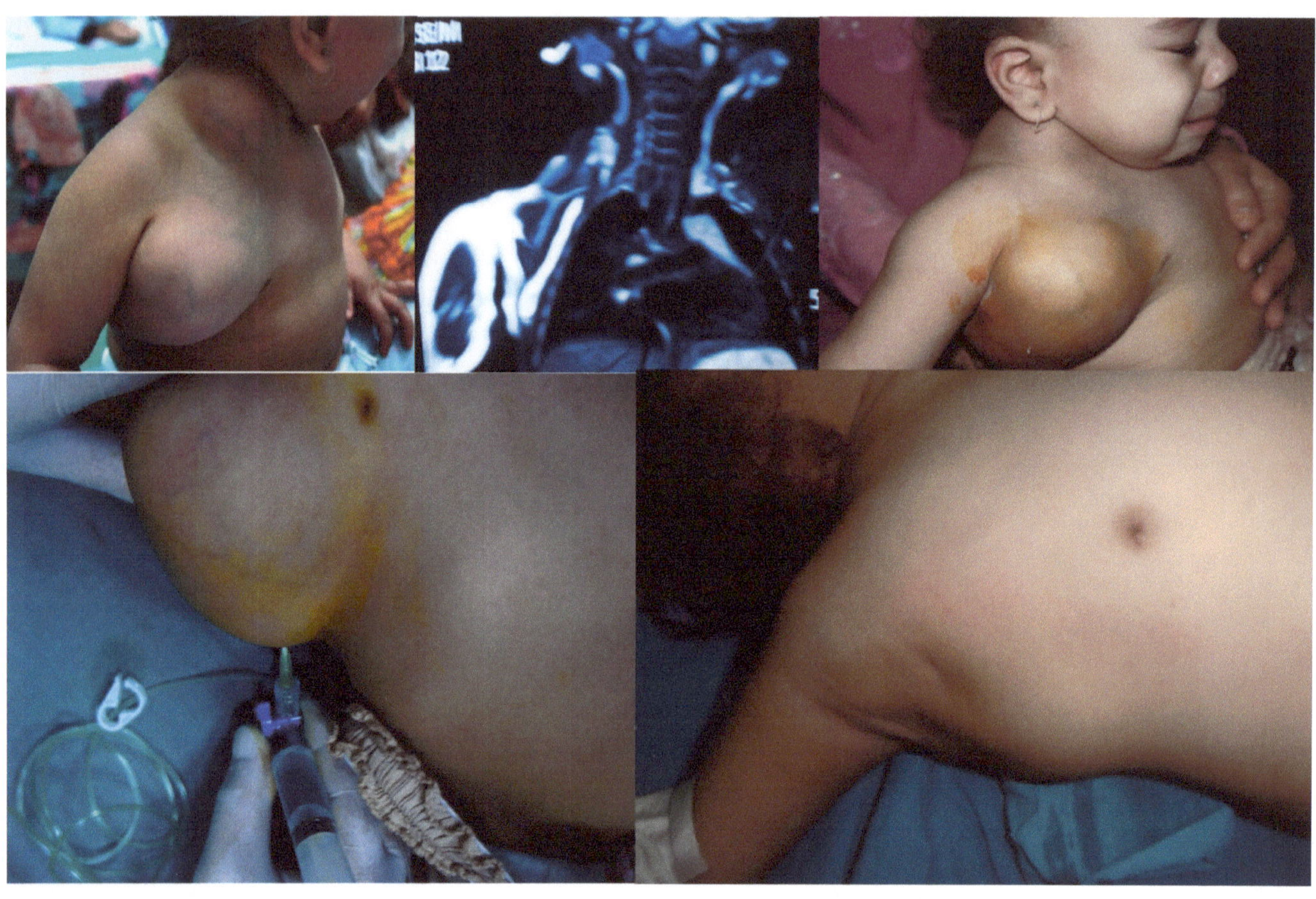

43.Submandibular cystic hygroma excised surgically

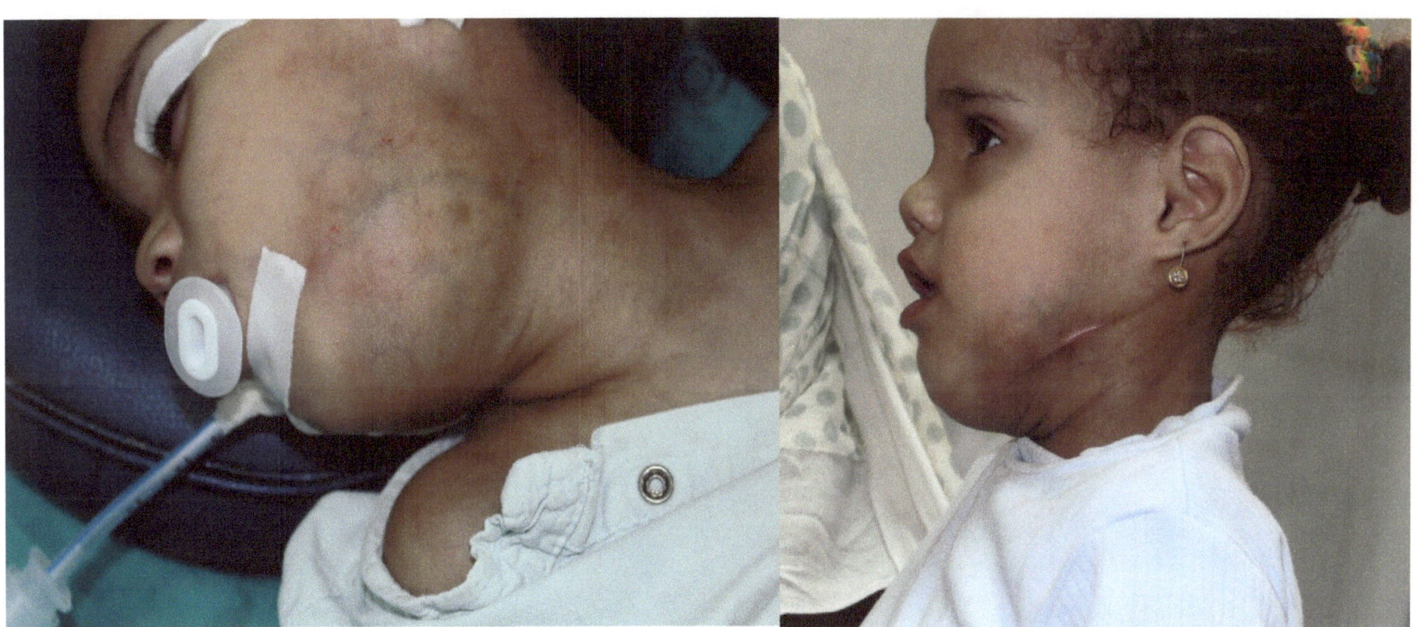

44.Huge thigh lymphatic malformation excised surgically

52

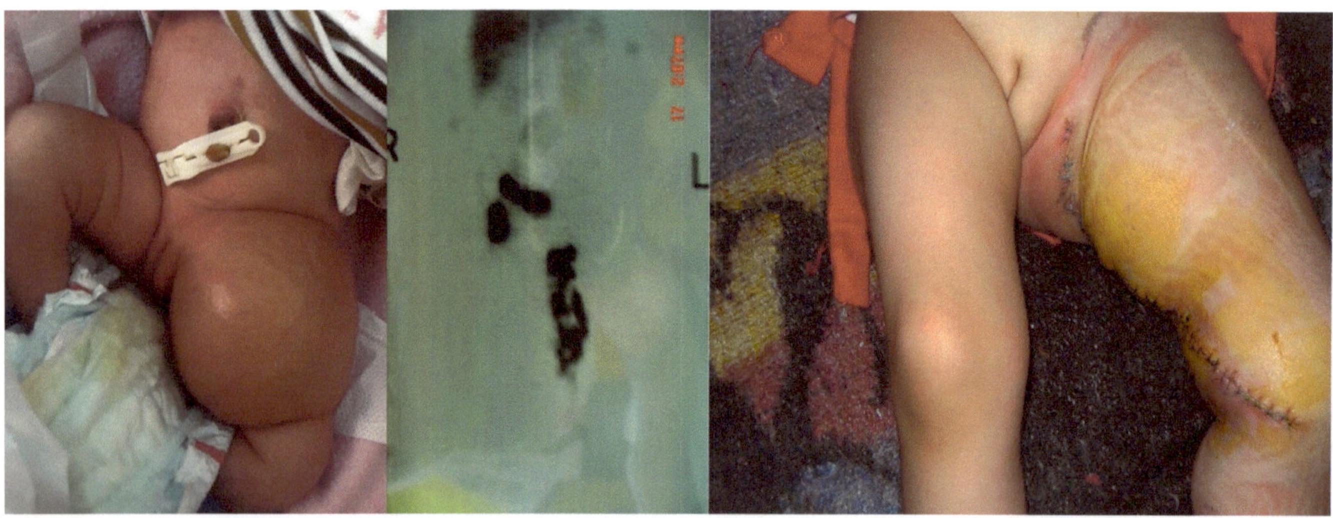

45. Huge combined axillary lymphatic and hygrometers malformation excised
    surgically

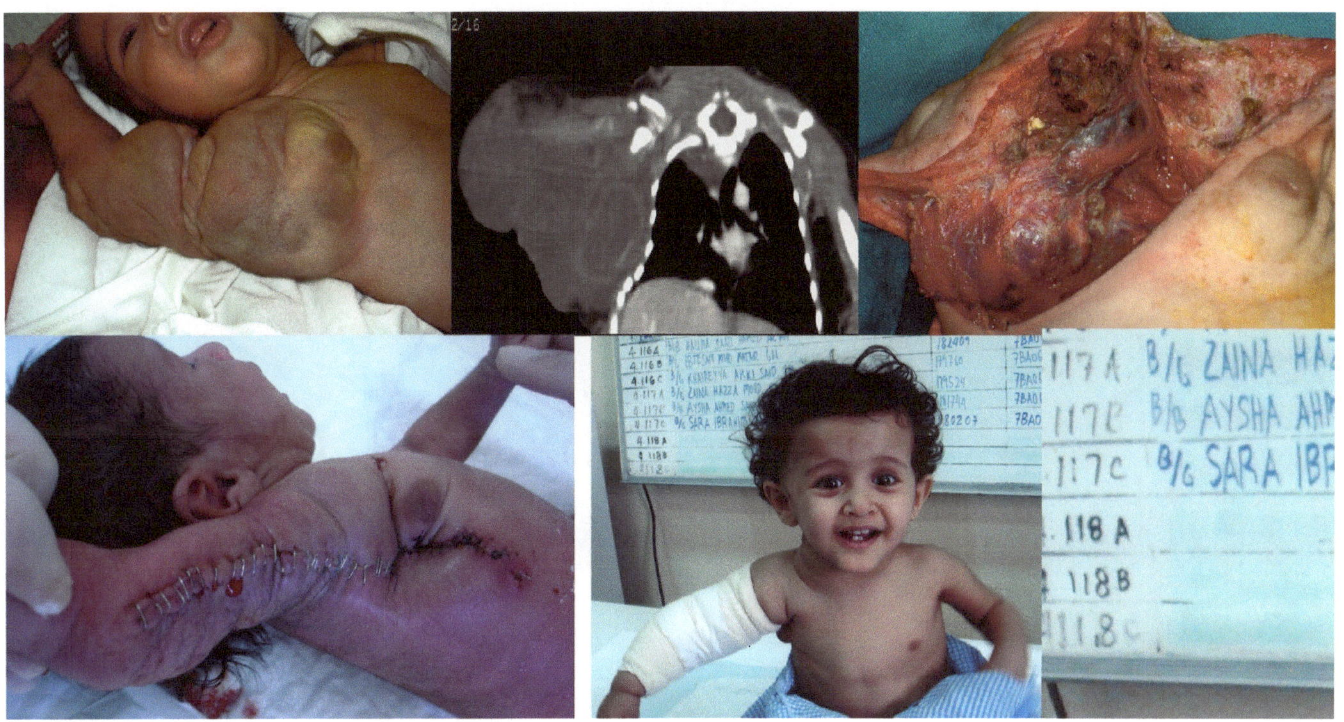

46. Different complications of bleomycin injection for the lymphatic
malformations

- Infection
- Non responding
- Ulceration

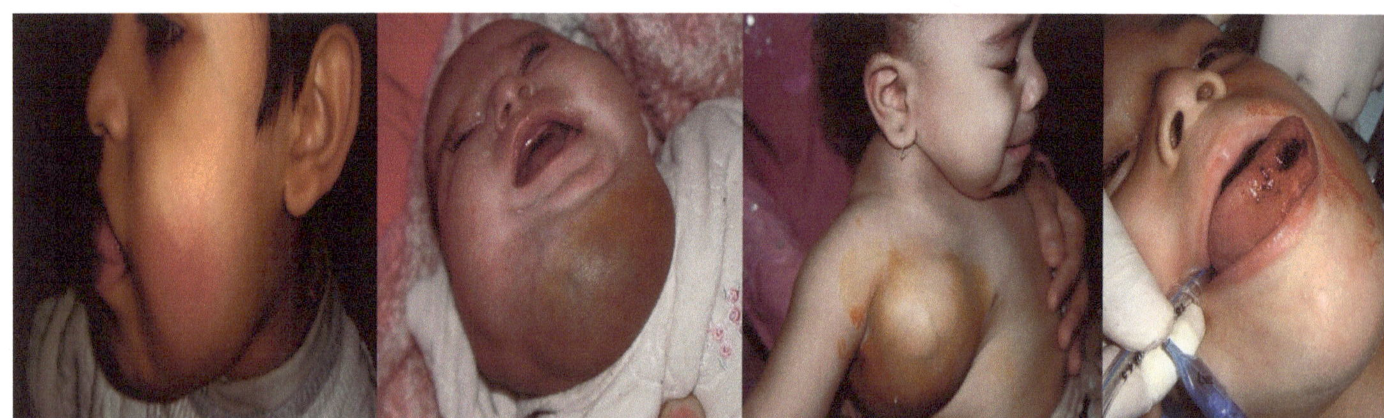

www.ingramcontent.com/pod-product-compliance
Lightning Source LLC
Chambersburg PA
CBHW040047240726
48664CB00004B/1100